Your Hidden Food Allergies Are Making You Fat

For more information on the ALCAT Test, please contact

AMTL Corporation
American Medical Testing Laboratories
One Oakwood Blvd., Suite 130
Hollywood, FL 33020
Tel.: (954) 923-2990 or (800) 881-2685
Fax: (954) 923-2707
http://www.alcat.com

Your Hidden Food Allergies Are Making You Fat

RUDY RIVERA, M.D., AND
ROGER DEUTSCH

PRIMA HEALTH

A Division of Prima Publishing

Library of Congress Cataloging-in-Publication Data
Rivera, Rudy
    Your hidden food allergies are making you fat : the ALCAT food sensitivities weight loss breakthrough / Rudy Rivera and Roger D. Deutsch
      p. cm.
    Includes bibliographical references and index.
    ISBN 0-7615-1434-1
    1. Food allergy—Complications. 2. Weight loss. 3. Obesity—Etiology.
    4. Blood—Examination. I. Deutsch, Roger D. II. Title.
    RC596.R68   1998
    616.97'5—dc21   98-25791
                                                                   CIP

98 99 00 01 HH 10 9 8 7 6 5 4 3 2 1
Printed in the United States of America

How to Order
Single copies may be ordered from Prima Publishing, P.O. Box 1260BK, Rocklin, CA 95677; telephone (916) 632-4400. Quantity discounts are also available. On your letterhead, include information concerning the in-tended use of the books and the number of books you wish to purchase.

Visit us online at www.primahealth.com

Dedicated to my loving wife
whose memory keeps me dreaming against all odds.
And to my two sons and daughter
who gave up their time with me
so this book could be written.

—RUDY RIVERA

This book is dedicated to my virtuous wife, Jenifer,
my strong and independent son, Jason,
and to my very best friends, R. and K.

—ROGER DEUTSCH

CONTENTS

Contents

CHAPTER 1

A Medical Breakthrough for the Twenty-first Century

I've tried all kinds of diets and I never kept the weight off. Now I'm losing weight without being hungry. I don't know how this is working, but it's working.

—Diane, housewife, Florida

The insulin dosage for my diabetes dropped from 90 to 20 units within one week.

—Joan, high school teacher, California

My panic disorder cleared up completely.

—Rose, registered nurse, Florida

Every season, I used to be constantly sick and struggle with colds and flu. Now, I'm totally healthy in spite of a big flu that got half our team.

—Christian Mayer, World Cup Winner,
Austrian Ski Team, Salzburg

> I lost about one-and-a-half pounds each week without chang-
> ing my activity level or consciously reducing portions. I
> found I wasn't as hungry and had fewer cravings.
>
> —John Magauran, M.D., general practitioner, Honolulu, Hawaii

How were these people able to achieve the optimum health and ideal weight that eludes so many of us today? What miracle pill or treatment transported them from a life of excess weight, physical pain, or mental distress to a life of maximum health and normal weight?

Proper diagnosis of food intolerance, a common but frequently ignored medical condition, made the difference in the lives of these five people—and thousands of others around the world. In fact, a proper diagnosis of food intolerance (also called food allergy and food sensitivity) is helping to cure a wide range of health-care problems from obesity to depression to diabetes. When you remove the specific foods that disturb your body's unique biochemistry, you are able to heal and operate at peak performance without nagging, even life-threatening symptoms. According to medical experts, recognizing and treating food intolerance may be just the medical breakthrough needed to treat the growing number of health problems that plague modern man. Here are a few of many comments made by doctors who have treated illness by showing their patients what foods are making them sick.

> Food intolerance and allergy have become an increasingly
> serious problem in recent decades. Food allergy might be
> the cause or aggravation of almost any disorder, and, often
> enough, it is *the* cause.
>
> —James C. Breneman, M.D., *Basics of Food Allergy*

It's a great disappointment that doctors don't bother to consider food intolerance, because removing certain foods from certain people's diets can be helpful with so many problems.

—John W. Gerrard, M.D., former professor of pediatrics,
University of Saskatchewan, Canada

Failure to recognize and control food allergy throughout life accounts for much unnecessary morbidity, invalidism, and even mortality.

—Albert H. Rowe, M.D., *Food Allergy: Its Manifestation and Control*

A New View of Food

At 56, Joan was dying. Her diabetes was out of control and she was 72 pounds overweight. No drug, diet, or therapy had any impact on her deteriorating health. One of her sisters had recently died from multiple sclerosis, and Joan's husband didn't want to lose his wife at such a young age. He insisted that she immediately go to the hospital for intensive medical attention. Joan said she trusted only one doctor with her life, so she flew across the country from San Francisco to Baltimore for an appointment with Dr. Barbara Solomon, a relative. Upon reviewing Joan's condition, Dr. Solomon suspected that food intolerance was contributing to her health problems. She explained that Joan's body was quite possibly reacting with hostility to common, otherwise "healthy" foods. Dr. Solomon immediately ordered a simple blood test to find out whether this was the case and, if so, exactly which foods were aggravating Joan's diabetes and obesity.

Within two days Joan learned something that completely surprised her—foods she ate every day were killing her. In fact, her body's biochemistry was reacting adversely to nearly 50 out of 100 common foods, including olives, nuts, wheat, certain fruits, white sugar, domesticated meats, and some types of fish. Although she did not understand how these wholesome foods could be making her sick, Joan nonetheless followed the doctor's orders and eliminated from her diet all her "allergenic" foods. She was stunned when her insulin requirement dropped from 90 units a day to 25 units within one week—an "extraordinary and life-saving change . . . nothing short of a miracle," according to Dr. Solomon.

What's more, within six months of removing her reactive foods from her diet, Joan, who stands five-feet-four-inches, lost 37 pounds—dropping from a dangerous 192 pounds to a comfortable 156. Despite the fact that her family had always eaten a healthy diet—including organic foods from the health-food store, fresh herbs from the family garden, and fruit from their own trees—once she stopped eating her intolerant foods, Joan felt better than she had in years. "My mood swings have disappeared, I handle stress better, I have more self-esteem, and I have more energy in my personal life and teaching career. I have even become more faithful with exercise, whereas previously I would choose a good book on the couch over a walk to the park. I can't say enough about the food intolerance test. I don't even want to think about where I'd be today without it."

The Key to Maximum Health and Minimum Weight

The diagnosis that literally saved Joan's life—food intolerance—has already helped improve the health of hundreds of thousands of other people around the world who suffer from a wide range of symptoms and illnesses, including diabetes, arthritis, obesity, chronic fatigue, migraines, panic attacks, intestinal problems, and childhood illnesses such as ear infections, attention deficit disorder, and bed-wetting. Food intolerance is not a medical diagnosis you hear every day—yet it's more common than most of us (including many medical professionals) realize. Although a complex biological process, food intolerance is, simply stated, an individualized biochemical sensitivity to foods that are otherwise wholesome and harmless. This sensitivity causes the immune system to react as if it were protecting the body from an enemy such as a bacteria, virus, or parasite. This reaction to common foods causes intricate systems within the body to begin malfunctioning. One abnormal function triggers and impacts the next, like a series of dominos falling, until the slow dance of dysfunction surfaces in one form of ill health or another.

This series of malfunctions begins when a person eats his or her intolerant foods. Usually protein molecules, or one or more chemicals (either naturally occurring or man-made) in these particular foods, cause a complex series of reactions, which eventually cause the white blood cells to react, and sometimes "explode." When they explode they release packets of chemicals that go to work to defend the body against the "invader." If these powerful chemicals have too many enemies to fight (the result of regularly eating your reactive foods), they can leave a trail of destruction. Several adverse reactions can result, such as leaky blood vessels, increased production of mucous, chronic inflammation of tissue, contraction of the smooth muscle of the lungs, intestines, and stomach, and general disruption of biochemical processes. These side effects can wreak havoc in the body, eventually impacting almost any organ and bringing about almost any disease and disease symptom. Like our fingerprints, none of our food sensitivities are the same (except by chance). While one person can eat all the chicken he wants without adverse effects, another might break out in hives the next day, develop a migraine two days later, or land in the hospital if she eats so much as a drumstick.

Your Own Personal Poison

Many of us confuse food intolerance with food allergy. Although the difference between the two is complicated, a simple distinction is that the person allergic to foods, such as peanuts, strawberries, or shrimp, reacts immediately—often with a rash or, in extreme cases, anaphylactic shock (a severe and sometimes fatal allergic response). This type of reaction to food is rare—less than five percent of the U.S. population exhibits what is called "true" food allergy. Food intolerance, on the other hand, is often referred to as the "hidden" food allergy, since you usually have no apparent immediate reaction when you eat a food to which your body is sensitive. In fact, our body's reaction to offending foods usually occurs in small steps. Each step leads to the next until at some point, the body reaches a breaking point—the final straw.

Our body then reacts by developing one or more of a wide range of symptoms and diseases such as obesity, arthritis, diabetes, gastrointestinal problems, sinus conditions, or migraines. The cellular changes may be so subtle and discrete that it is impossible for us to associate them with a food eaten regularly; yet continuing to eat this food will progressively deteriorate our physical health. Doctors who understand the profound relationship between food and health, and who understand and respect the destructive forces of food intolerance, can offer us relief. No drug, no medical therapy, and no diet alone can improve your health or help you lose weight if you continue to bombard your body with your own personal poison.

Joan and other sufferers who struggle for maximum health and normal weight (and sometimes for their lives) have learned that food intolerance is indeed their health problem—or an important part of their problem. For unlike the rarely occurring food allergy, food intolerance is common. Current research from a variety of sources estimates that between 30 and 90 percent of the general population suffers from food intolerance, which may manifest as relatively mild acne or a stuffy nose to conditions as deadly as diabetes or asthma. Growing evidence demonstrates that food intolerance may also play a significant role in the greatest health epidemic faced by the medical community today—obesity. As the correlation between biochemistry and overweight becomes increasingly apparent, it's not surprising that intolerance to foods contributes to the biological glitch that makes so many of us too fat for our own good health.

No drug, no medical therapy, and no diet alone can improve your health or help you lose weight if you continue to bombard your body with your own personal poison.

Like Joan, we find it hard to believe that otherwise healthful foods could contribute to health problems. After all, most of us were raised to believe that good foods build strong bones, enrich blood, and keep the doctor away. It seems illogical that a glass of fresh milk, iron-rich beef, or an innocent apple has the potential to make us sick. Yet when Walter drinks milk, he develops severe gastrointestinal problems; when Barbara eats a hamburger, she gets a migraine; and when Sue eats even a little bit of apple, her eczema returns. Often, people don't believe the reality of food intolerance until they see the impact in their own lives.

Arthritis Sufferer Finds a Simple Cure

Carla first heard about food intolerance in the office of Dr. Jay Sandweiss, an internist in Detroit. Sandweiss was on the long list of doctors she'd seen in her desperate search to find relief from worsening arthritis. During Carla's first office visit, Dr. Sandweiss recommended the ALCAT Test for food and chemical intolerance. When the test results showed that Carla was intolerant to chocolate and green beans, she thought she had wasted her money again. She left the office feeling let down by yet another medical practitioner. Dr. Sandweiss didn't hear from Carla again until a year later when she wrote to explain that she'd thought he was a quack when he recommended the food intolerance test. Then, when he told her she was allergic to common foods and that they were contributing to her worsening arthritis, she was *sure* he was giving her a bunch of baloney. But one day she thought:

> Well, I've spent the money, I might as well try eliminating
> these foods and see what happens. And to my amazement
> my arthritis went away. I had no pain, and I was able to do
> needlepoint and all the things I hadn't done in years. Then
> I got overconfident and ate some chocolate at Christmas.
> When I woke up the next day I was crippled in pain again.
> Now I keep my diet cleaned of all my reactive foods and I'm
> totally cured. You changed my life and I can't believe the
> food I was eating is what was causing my health problem.

Food Intolerance Saves the Day . . . and a Life

No one has to tell Sharon how insidious food intolerance can be at destroying health. After eating a bit of salad one day, the chronic stomach pains she'd had for years—cramps, bloating, and gas—escalated to the point of panic. Her stomach hurt so badly she thought she was going to die of a diseased colon—as her father had six months prior. "My health was deteriorating so rapidly that I was sure I was next," she remembers. A gastrointestinal specialist performed a test and found that her entire colon was inflamed and covered in ulcers and polyps. He put her on medication, which turned her skin yellow and made her feel worse.

As luck would have it, a dietitian she was seeing at the time to help her lose weight recommended she be tested for food intolerance. The test showed that Sharon had many food sensitivities—so many in fact, that she was left with only a few foods to eat, including turkey, lamb, tuna, squash, and spinach. Desperate to try anything that might make the excruciating pain go away, she embarked on her specially designed diet, which eliminated all her intolerant foods. On the tenth day she felt like a new person. "I'll remember that day as long as I live—it was a euphoric feeling," says Sharon. "I immediately called my doctor to tell him that I felt better and was going off the pills. He scheduled a check-up right away. He was shocked to find my colon as healthy as any he'd ever seen. All the inflammation, ulcers, and polyps were gone. The food intolerance test saved my life. I would recommend this test for anyone and everyone."

Free from a Prison of Fat

The problem of obesity is so great in our nation that major health-care organizations are scrambling to find an effective and healthy way to deal with what's been called "the fattening of America." Much current research on weight loss points solidly in the direction of a correlation between obesity and a biochemical glitch in the brain—a similar biological glitch to that created by food intolerance. Research already shows that people not only lose weight on a diet that eliminates their intolerant foods, but they lose *fat,* not lean muscle.

While research clearly shows that eliminating intolerant foods from the diet is an effective weight-loss approach, the greatest proof lies in personal stories of triumph over conditions that were ruining lives by trapping people in prisons of fat. Dianna's story has been repeated by thousands of weight watchers around the world. For years, Dianna had struggled with her weight, losing and gaining the same 30 pounds many times. She'd tried every popular diet and none were helping her lose and keep off weight. Eventually she found herself 60 pounds overweight and feeling out of control. Fortunately, she met up with an old friend who had also struggled with weight. "She had lost so much weight that she looked like she'd lost another person," says Dianna. "I barely recognized her. I asked her how she lost her weight and she told me about food intolerance. She had eliminated foods that her body didn't tolerate and ate all she wanted of everything else, and she lost weight for the first time in years. It sounded too good to be true."

Despite her disbelief, Dianna scheduled an appointment to have her blood tested for her food intolerances, and was surprised to learn that she was sensitive to many foods, including the very foods she was eating on her many weight-loss diets. Her new food-intolerant diet basically consisted of all she wanted of beef, chicken, fish, eggs, spinach, cabbage, beets, carrots, celery, lettuce, walnut oil, and some grains. Within seven months she'd lost all her excess weight. "I lost the weight slowly, and I wasn't hungry at all. I was completely satisfied with whatever I ate. I don't know why this diet worked when everything else failed. I'm afraid to even question it, but it worked."

Rose was another lucky overweight person who learned about food intolerance and finally conquered her battle with the bulge. She was 160 pounds overweight and had tried every diet on the market when she learned about food intolerance from a dietitian who had already helped many people lose weight. Rose had her blood tested and stopped eating her reactive foods, but ate as much as she wanted of every other food. She lost 100 pounds in six months and felt better than she had in years. "I have been on so many different diets over the years, but I felt different on this one. I felt very healthy and I had no food cravings. My energy level was intoxicating," Rose says. "I wished that I could bottle that energy and take a whiff every now and then."

World Class Health

More energy and better performance is something everyone craves in our modern world with its endless list of "to do's" and daily stresses. But the idea of better performance takes on a whole new meaning when you are a world-class athlete competing in major sporting events, where a fraction of a second can mean the difference between winning and losing. Just ask Christian Mayer, a skier with the Austrian Ski Team, who won the World Cup in the Giant Slalom two years in a row and a bronze medal at the Winter Olympics in Lillehammer.

Mayer went to see Austrian physician Dr. Stephen Schimpf at the suggestion of his team's coach when his chronic stuffy nose began to interfere with his performance. Dr. Schimpf immediately tested him for food intolerance and found several sensitivities, including to milk, wheat, tomatoes, and beer. After eliminating those foods, not only did Christian's stuffy nose disappear, but his headaches disappeared, he lost ten pounds of off-season excess weight, and he had greater energy. "After the diet I was much quicker in the slalom and felt much stronger overall; and best of all, I'm still winning," he says. "At the end of every season, I used to gain ten pounds. Now, with the framework of my food-intolerance food plan, I can eat what I want and I don't gain even one pound. Also, I used to be constantly sick and struggle with colds and flus. Now, I'm totally healthy in spite of a big flu that got half our team."

Dr. Schimpf has since tested other members of the Austrian ski team for their food intolerances as well as many other Austrian sportspeople. "They have all had extremely good results—they feel more energetic, keep off extra weight more easily, and perform better. In fact, many have gone public to explain the benefit they've received from the food intolerance testing. These Austrian athletes are absolutely convinced that knowing and avoiding their food intolerances is the way to improve their health and maximize their performance."

No Longer Sick and Tired

More energy and better performance is needed not just in the realm of world-class athletes. All of us need more energy to keep up with the demands of our modern world. And yet, more of us than ever suffer from chronic, low-grade symptoms that zap our energy and make even simple chores pile up like so much deadwood after a storm. From our mid-afternoon slumps to chronic fatigue syndrome, too many of us are tired these days for this condition to be a coincidence. Something is clearly wrong. But what?

Many practitioners point their fingers at food intolerance. Why?

Because when patients like Rose and Christian eliminate their intolerant foods they have more energy than they've had in years. Cleason, another example, could not seem to regain his strength after two bouts with the flu. He became so tired that he missed days of work, then finally stopped going to work altogether. Luckily, his wife had learned about food intolerance when seeking a cure for her children's health problems. Cleason had tried many therapies suggested by several doctors, but it wasn't until he removed his intolerant foods that he lost the excessive tiredness, regained his energy, and was able to return to work.

Spared a Lifetime of Illness

The diagnosis of food intolerance has helped not only adults; children also benefit from learning which foods and other substances, such as dyes and preservatives, cause adverse reactions in their bodies. A long list of children's health problems, including ear infections, hyperactivity/ attention deficit disorder (ADHD), autism, headaches, and eczema can be linked to food intolerance. Dozens of research studies show how removing children's intolerant foods (and food chemicals) can improve their health, and even cure debilitating conditions. Dr. Walter Ward, an ear, nose, and throat/allergy specialist in North Carolina, says that one of the most dramatic medical cases he's ever encountered involved a boy of five, whose mother had brought him in for sinus problems. The child also had severe renal problems, which physicians at a highly respected hospital were trying in vain to treat. "Those medical professionals were following traditional renal therapy, but it was having no impact," says Dr. Ward. "The kidneys were just going, and the doctors were essentially watching the kid die." He consulted a colleague from the University of Miami, who recommended the ALCAT Test. The child went off his reactive foods and his health immediately took an upward turn. Within a short time his kidneys were functioning normally.

Breakthrough Medical Treatment

These are only a few of thousands of stories about people who turned their health around, even saved their lives, by knowing and eliminating their food intolerances. If food intolerance testing can help the Joannas, Carlas, Roses, Christians, and Cleasons of the world improve their health, then food intolerance testing may very likely be the breakthrough medical treatment of the twenty-first century. Especially when you consider the billions of dollars already spent on research, medical technology developments, increasingly complex surgical treatments, and pharmaceutical creations, it's shocking that we are sicker and fatter than ever. In the U.S. alone, 12 million suffer from diabetes, 16 million from arthritis, and 50 percent of the country's adults are overweight. And that's just the tip of the iceberg. The health of increasing numbers of people worldwide is being compromised by medical treatments that aren't working. All the while, the answer to maximum health and healthy weight may be as near as your kitchen table. Stop eating the foods that overload your system and cause your body to attack the foreigners, and you'll enjoy optimum health.

It's almost too simple to believe. Further good news is this: Unlike "trying" prescription drugs, surgeries, or other therapies, and dealing with the often-severe side effects, eliminating your reactive foods and seeing what happens poses no risk to your health whatsoever. Like Rose and Dianna, you may lose your excess weight and gain energy. Like Cleason and Carla, you may recover from illnesses that crippled your ability to live life to the fullest. Or like Joan and Sharon, you may find the cure to the chronic illness that not only forces you to live life in poor health, but is leading you to premature death.

Food intolerance testing and treatment is a simple, painless, nonsurgical, nonpharmaceutical approach to improving health. By properly diagnosing our food sensitivities, the impact on the health, health-care costs, mortality, and quality of life of our nation's citizens could be truly profound. It could be just what an ailing society needs to live productive, happy, and healthy lives in what's sure to be an exciting and challenging twenty-first century.

Diagnosis: Food Intolerance

According to current researchers in this area, anywhere from 30 to 90 percent of the population of the United States is intolerant of one or more foods. This number is believed to be rising due to several lifestyle factors in the modern world. The health implications of food intolerance vary widely. While your symptoms may be as relatively minor as a runny nose, your neighbor may have crippling arthritis, and your relative may be chronically overweight. Whether you live a life of minor, but chronic, health problems that only inconvenience your lifestyle, or you suffer from a health problem that is developing into a life-threatening disease, or if you're somewhere between these extremes, you should find out whether food intolerance is the culprit.

A new technology can identify the exact foods that may be causing a person to be sick and/or overweight. This patented technology is a simple computerized blood test, which measures any changes to white blood cells in the presence of common foods. If the white blood cells become enlarged, burst, or shrink, these changes set the stage for serious health problems that develop immediately or perhaps years later.

If you're living a life of glowing health, unencumbered by any health problems, you may be among the lucky few who do not have an aberrant biochemical reaction to any food or food chemical. But it's time to find out whether common foods are causing or exacerbating your health woes and to avoid those foods if one or more of the following symptoms have become a permanent fixture in your life:

Acne	Ear infections
Anxiety	Eczema
Arthritis	Fatigue
Asthma	Hay fever
Attention deficit hyper-activity disorder (ADHD)	Headaches (tension type and migraine)
Autism	Inflammatory bowel disease
Bed-wetting	Muscle aches
Chronic diarrhea	Obesity
Chronic fatigue	Panic attacks
Depression	Stuffy nose
Diabetes	Urticaria

Although these are the most common food intolerance symptoms, food intolerance has been implicated in nearly any symptom imaginable. Unlike many medical conditions, which either test positive or negative (such as heart disease, hepatitis, and cancer), food intolerance manifests in a wide range of degrees. What's more, it fluctuates. Sometimes a food-intolerant person will have a good day and be symptom-free, and other days he or she will be totally incapacitated by ill health.

Evolution of a Valid Testing Method

Though it has long been known that reactions to foods can cause many unpleasant symptoms, the vast numbers of foods present in our diets complicate treatment. Once it was recognized that food sensitivities are caused by multiple factors, the white blood cells seemed a logical place to look for change. Because the white blood cell population is a final common pathway of all the various pathogenic mechanisms, a test was needed to detect specific changes in these white blood cells that would identify a specific food as reactive.

Food intolerance testing and treatment is a simple, painless, nonsurgical, nonpharmaceutical approach to improving health.

In the 1930s Drs. Robert Cooke and Warren T. Vaughn developed a method for testing food sensitivities. They withdrew blood from the subject and, using the methods available at the time, counted the white blood cells. They then had the subject eat the food in question. Some time after ingestion of the food, blood was withdrawn for the second time and the white blood cells counted again. If the counts were appreciably lower, the food was considered reactive. Cooke and Vaughn's method was dubbed the "Leucocytopenic Index."

Following from this, in the mid-1950s an allergist in El Paso named Arthur Black published his work studying changes in white blood cells challenged with an allergen and then viewed under a microscope. He observed that some allergens caused the white cells to disintegrate and release chemical mediators of inflammation. These allergens were confirmed to cause clinical symptoms in many cases. A husband and wife team, William and Mary Bryan from Washington University, later took up this work and this "cytoxic" test became quite popular for some time. However, this test was never really accepted by mainstream medicine because, it was argued, the results were subjective and not easily reproduced. Some feel the test was not given a fair evaluation because it posed a serious threat to the status quo in medical practice.

Around 1983, American Medical Testing Laboratories began research on an automated and objective method for measuring changes in white blood cells and other cells when the blood is exposed to a battery of test substances. Foods were the primary focus, though food colorings, food additives, environmental chemicals, certain drugs, and other substances can be tested as well. The test, named the ALCAT Test,* uses a specially designed hematology analyzer with results that are interpreted by a computer. This renders the test objective and reproducible. Scientific research has validated the method (see page 285). Physicians' offices can request reprints of numerous studies at no cost by contacting this address:

---

*The name ALCAT was originally an acronym for the Antigen Leukocyte Cellular Antibody Test. The ALCAT Test has changed dramatically and now measures a much broader range of reactions than the original test; however, the acronym was retained.

American Medical Testing Laboratories
One Oakwood Blvd., Suite 130
Hollywood, FL 33020
Phone: (954) 923-2990
  (800) 881-AMTL
Fax: (954) 923-2707
Web site: www.alcat.com.

What You Should Know about Food Intolerance

This book will give you the most comprehensive look at this astounding medical condition too long overlooked by medicine practitioners. To help you understand food intolerance and its possible impact on you and your children's health and weight, the following chapters will explore:

- the breakthrough study on the impact of food intolerance on weight and health
- the field of food intolerance including what causes it
- how common foods can impact your body and deteriorate your health
- why you may not be aware of this condition
- the details of treating several modern health-care problems such as obesity and chronic fatigue through food intolerance
- how a simple blood test can tell you within a few days exactly which foods and food chemicals your system cannot tolerate
- the stories of dozens of people whose lives are already brimming with good health because they learned about their food intolerances
- how you can get on the road to maximum health and healthy weight

You'll learn how to help your body adapt to the challenges of our modern world—and how a simple technology has finally been developed to deal with twentieth-century health problems. Follow in the footsteps of thousands who have already learned that the foods they eat every day are preventing their enjoying a life of optimal health. Discover and manage your food intolerances and you, too, may finally experience the maximum health and normal weight you desire.

CHAPTER 2

Overweight: The Plague of Our Age

Without our ability to gain weight, humans as a species would never survive. In the world of our prehistoric ancestors, the hunters and gatherers, food was not always plentiful. When berries and roots were in season and when wild animals were not hibernating, our ancestors ate well—and they fattened up. Then during seasons when food was harder to come by, they relied on their stored fat to see them through the lean times.

Two biological functions assisted them as they struggled to survive this perpetual cycle of feasts and famines. When they had abundant food, their bodies efficiently stored fat, and during times when there was less to eat, their metabolism slowed to adjust to the smaller quantities of food. They were genetically programmed to adapt their metabolic rates to food intake. Those who survived were blessed with "fat-storing" genes, while those who lacked these genes perished. And the survivors passed their "thrifty" genes on to future generations—in other words, to us. These genes, which evolve slowly over thousands of generations, have not caught up to modern living and eating. We use the same genes to program our bodies to store concentrated sugars, processed carbohydrates, and adulterated fats.

Prehistoric Bodies
in the Modern Western World

Ironically, the same biological self-preservation mechanism that helped our ancestors store and retain fat—and thereby survive cycles of feast and famine—is one of the factors ruining our health, even killing some of us today. Thousands die each year from health problems related to obesity (an estimated 300,000 people died in 1990 alone, according to a congressional report). Further, obesity is a contributing risk factor for four of the seven leading causes of death. Former U.S. Surgeon General C. Everett Koop stated that obesity is the second greatest preventable cause of death, right behind smoking. In his 1994 "Shape Up America" campaign report, Koop stated that excess weight is "one of the most pervasive health threats affecting Americans today." What's more, obesity is on the rise more than ever before in our history. According to Dr. Philip James, a leading Scottish authority on nutrition and chairman of an international task force on obesity, "Obesity is doubling every five years so we have an epidemic that is coming at the health service like a tidal wave."

Current statistics appear to confirm Dr. James's prediction. In 1996, a Department of Agriculture study revealed that at least 33 percent of all adults in the United States are overweight (more than 20 percent above their ideal body weight). That figure is up from the 25 percent reported just ten years ago. Other calculations are even more grim: According to a 1995 report by the Institute of Medicine, 59 percent of the adult population meets the current definition of clinical obesity, which qualifies the disease for epidemic status. Adults aren't the only ones suffering from excess weight. A recently released Surgeon General's report says more children ages 12 to 20 are more overweight than ever before. According to the National Center for Health Statistics, one in every five children in the U.S. is considered overweight. It's no wonder the Institute of Medicine has declared war on the nation's "epidemic of obesity."

The Plague of Our Age

Why is the genetic self-preservation system we inherited from our prehistoric ancestors failing us in our modern world? One reason is that an important part of the feast and famine cycle is missing from the lifestyle of Western and developed societies—the famines, which resulted in mandatory food fasts. No longer do we struggle through periods with very little food—thanks to modern food farming, preservation, storage, shipping, and preparation methods. On the contrary, we live in a perpetual feast— eating seasonal foods all year long, consuming exotic foods grown around the world and shipped to our neighborhood grocery, and indulging in every conceivable convenience food that food manufacturers can dream up. This means that our bodies are always on "store" mode. Rarely are they on use-up-the-excess-fuel mode—except, of course, when we go on low-fat diets in our perpetual, mostly hopeless, effort to lose excess weight. As most dieters now realize, this sets the body up to eventually cycle back around to nature's uncontrollable call to eat. The sad fact is that the body, as soon as possible after a "diet" (which the body interprets as a famine and therefore a threat), reacts by quickly regaining the lost weight—and more—in preparation for the next food shortage, just as it did for our prehistoric ancestors.

An August 1996 article in *Scientific American* sums up our modern predicament well, stating that our growing problem of obesity can be blamed on "exceptionally thrifty genes—turned loose in an environment that offers easy access to high-energy food while requiring little hard labor." This brings us to another reason for America's excess of "saddlebags" and "spare tires." While our ancestors had to work for their supper (from chasing down tigers to raising chickens), modern man can enjoy three meals a day plus snacks while exerting very little energy. F. Xavier PiSunyer, director of the Obesity Research Center at St. Luke's–Roosevelt Hospital in New York City, predicted in the same article, "we are going to see a continuing increase in obesity over the next 25 years" as standards of living continue to rise. Genetic heritage, too much food, and not enough exercise are among the many reasons why modern man in industrialized nations is facing the obesity plague. But one more reason is just now becoming clear to a growing number of health-care practitioners— food intolerance contributes to the increasing problem of overweight, and the modern world "feast" is causing more people to develop food intolerances.

Fatter Than Ever . . .

There are many reasons why we are fatter than ever before. The modern Western diet consists largely of over-processed, fatty foods manufactured by the ever-expanding food industry. These are known as "skeletonized" foods. With all or most of their nutrients removed by processing, they are little more than fat and carbohydrate skeletons of their original form.

Also, we live increasingly sedentary lifestyles, thanks in large part to modern technology. And the increasing prevalence of food intolerance is causing vast numbers of biological malfunctions that result in internal disturbances such as inappropriate fat storage, inefficient use of the stored fat, food cravings, and water retention.

A 1996 article in *Obesity Research* sums up the problem of obesity this way: "[The] modern Western lifestyle appears to provide the social and emotional conditions that favor maximum expression of underlying individual genetic differences in susceptibility to overweight." What this means is that our twentieth-century Western lifestyle—with its highly processed foods, chemicals, pollution, stress, industrialization, and social structure—is triggering and exacerbating the body's instinct to prepare for and defend against famine. Today's lifestyle has wreaked havoc in the people who inherently have a genetic propensity to gain excess weight—which, statistically, includes most of us. This is an important viewpoint.

Experts at a 1996 World Health Organization (WHO) conference said that the worldwide trend toward fatter people is due in part to the increase of machines, which lead to a more sedentary lifestyle. They added that the human brain biochemistry of modern man has not been able to adapt quickly enough to the reduced need for calories in our more sedentary lives, and that people are still eating as if they plowed farmland and milked cows for ten hours every day. Studies cited by the WHO task force showed that with the many different populations around the world getting fatter, experts are dealing with a complicated environmental problem that needs an environmental solution. In June 1998 Karen Donato of the National Institute of Health said: "According to the most recent national survey data, about 55 percent of American adults are overweight or obese—up from 43 percent in 1960." In this Associated Press release, Ms. Donato points out that "People eat out often. Portion sizes are larger than ever." And as a nation we spend "too much time sitting at our computers, driving the car, watching TV and taking the elevator instead of the stairs."

. . . And Getting Fatter

Fat on the body is not, in and of itself, unhealthy. On the contrary, we all need some fat to keep us warm and provide a cushion for our bones and organs. Only when fat grows to excess do we have a problem. Excess fat is uncomfortable, unhealthy, and deemed by society as unattractive. And as current research points out, obesity is more unhealthy than we ever realized.

Obesity, as mentioned above, currently affects at least one-third of the American population. But researchers fear that it's rising at an alarming rate. One study predicted that if obesity continues to increase at its current rate, every single man, woman, and child will be obese by the year 2030. Doctors who met at an international congress in Barcelona in 1996 said that obesity, with its often fatal complications, had become epidemic and could become a worldwide health disaster if not taken seriously and treated as a chronic disease.

One theory on the dramatic rise of obesity is that overweight people do not fully comprehend the health hazards of being overweight and therefore are not truly motivated to find an approach that will help them take off and keep off weight. However, the health hazards of obesity are serious and are now becoming fully understood. They include diabetes, heart disease, high blood pressure, high cholesterol levels, atherosclerosis, osteoarthritis, gallbladder disease, sleep apnea, weakened joints, and some forms of cancer. Research conducted by epidemiologists at Harvard University reported recently that being even 20 pounds overweight invited disease and poor health. In 1990 (the last year studied), epidemiologists at Harvard conservatively estimated that treating the ailments that result from obesity in the U.S. alone cost $45.8 billion, while indirect costs due to missed work added in another $23 billion. Experts of the WHO task force calculate that between 5 and 10 percent of the total health budgets of Western countries are involved with obesity, including treatment of the obesity-related illnesses such as arthritis, high blood pressure, back problems, and physiotherapy costs.

Beyond these serious health concerns, overweight people take a psychological beating from the social stigma of being overweight. Consider this commentary from a newspaper article written by a health writer from *The Boston Globe* regarding our nation's view of overweight people: "Americans have a curious relationship with fat. We're fat and getting fatter. Our eating habits are depraved, and our lifestyle is sedentary. We spend billions annually on diets and exercise programs and then don't stick to them. We turn to diet drugs. We resort to liposuction. We look to magazines for advice and find articles that warn of eating disorders alongside details of the latest semi-starvation diet, or 'eating plan' in the current argot. We hate fat. We fear fat. Fat people remind us of what we are, or what we could become if we're not careful. So we distance ourselves by making fun of them." Is it any wonder that obese people are 20 percent less likely to marry than their thinner counterparts? Research also shows that the household income of obese people is nearly $7,000 less than that of thinner people, and they are 10 percent more likely to live a life of poverty. All totaled, obesity and its ramifications have an obvious depressing effect on self-esteem.

Despite the desperate search underway to find an effective way to battle the bulge, all the current research on obesity is pointing to one fact: There is no magic bullet for losing excess weight. Obesity is a complex problem, which requires a change in our attitude about food and a change in the way we eat. But in which way do we change our eating habits? "Eating differently" is precisely what distinguishes various diets. Some claim that cutting calories is the ticket to melting the pounds away. Others claim low-fat diets will help you fit into your favorite pair of jeans. Still others point to high-protein diets as the path to slim-dom, and that's only a few of the options for the person who craves a life free from unsightly excess fat.

Yet the fact is that none of these approaches is working for the vast majority of the population. Although people do tend to lose weight on the programs, they also regain it over time. Recent clinical studies show that over 95 percent of people who use diets to control their weight gain it all back within five years. Dr. Claude Lenfant, director of the National Institute of Health's National Heart, Lung and Blood Institute, points out: "The difficulty lies in treating what is a very complex condition, affected by many social, cultural, behavioral, physiological, metabolic and genetic factors."

Fat and Unhappy

Although an estimated 55 percent of American adults are overweight, the percentage of people who are trying to lose weight is far greater. Their strategies range from over-the-counter diet pills to physician-supervised weight-loss programs that integrate exercise and dieting with psychological counseling. Unfortunately, most people who need to lose weight are not succeeding. And there is not much scientific evidence to indicate that any of these strategies is consistently effective for most people. But still we try.

Among the many methods that dieters employ in their determination to be slim and healthy are low-calorie diets. At any one time, headlines can be found in several newsstand publications proclaiming new weight-reduction diets and promising instant success: "Never Diet Again!" "Lose Weight Fast As You Walk!" "Blast Up to 49 Pounds Off in Only 29 Days!" The claims made by many so-called miracle weight-loss programs are indeed tempting. But few have any research or long-term success stories to back them up. On the contrary, science is providing an increasingly convincing body of evidence to explain why it is extremely difficult for many people to achieve and maintain their desired body weight through low-calorie diets. The fact is that these "miracle diets" are as effective as the snake oil sold by nineteenth century hucksters as a cure for everything from baldness to hemorrhoids.

A Billion-Dollar Industry on the Rise

Tempting claims like these are the reason the weight loss industry is a billion-dollar business—in fact, close to $30 billion in 1998. The 1998 sales of diet soft drinks is estimated at $12.5 billion, artificial sweeteners at $1.54 billion, health club memberships at $10 billion, commercial weight loss centers at $1 billion, low calorie foods at more than $2 billion, and appetite suppressants at $1 billion. Add to this books, tapes, seminars, doctor's office visits, and so forth, and the costs are staggering.

The weight-loss industry is not making money because its methods are working. It's making billions of dollars because it's *not* working. The same overweight person will try the same weight-loss program over and over, paying the often exorbitant rates for diet "secrets" until they finally give up and find a new diet program to spend their money on.

People repeatedly go on these "low-calorie weight-loss" diets with the blind faith that this time it will work; all they need is the willpower. They never stop to consider that the very premise of quick weight-loss diets is flawed—and that the only thing guaranteed in the long run is their failure. Statistically, when people lose weight on a low-calorie diet, they gain all the weight back within the first year. One reason that these diets are ineffective is because they are designed to have marketing sizzle, not practical guidance. After all, how many people would knock down the doors of weight-loss clinics if their advertisements said, "Lose one pound a week by eating healthy and sensibly and by exercising daily"? Such ads simply wouldn't fly in America. We want stupendous results and we want them *now*. So instead, the diet companies make claims such as "eat all you want" and "lose 10 pounds in 10 days."

The weight-loss industry is not making money because its methods are working. It's making billions of dollars because it's not working.

These ads recycle year after year, despite the fact that they don't work and despite the fact that they fly in the face of the reality of our body's actual biology. *Human Nutrition* gave this actual scientific description of how fat is gained or lost: "If energy intake and expenditure are not equally balanced, a deficit or excess of 3,500 kcal (kilo calories) normally causes a loss or gain of 1 pound of body fat. So, to result in weight loss, a person's food intake and activity level must cause energy expenditure to be 3,500 kcal greater than energy intake for every pound of weight loss."

This description is something most dieters have heard before, right? Eliminate the magic 3,500 calories and a pound of fat will melt off. Well, listen to this additional, rarely discussed, explanation of weight loss from Gilbert Kaats, Ph.D.: "These figures assume that *stored body fat* is the source of the energy needed to make up for the deficit, which is the case in people who are overweight or obese. If muscle or other fat-free mass is being broken down to supply energy, however, then a deficit of only 580 kcal results in a loss of 1 pound of weight. This reflects the lower energy content of fat-free tissue, which is 70% water. Loss of fat-free tissue produces the weight loss seen in starvation or severe malnutrition. Muscle loss is undesirable and in fact dangerous if there is appreciable loss, especially because it can affect the vital muscles of the heart."

Did you catch the significance of this explanation? It takes a deficit of 3,500 kcal to lose one pound of fat and only a mere 580 kcal to lose one pound of muscle, which is mostly water. So, if you've ever lost weight quickly on a low-calorie diet, what you've actually lost is muscle and water—not fat! This is no small fact. You may feel great when you look at the scale after a quick weight-loss diet, but in the long run you will have done more damage than good. Even though you have lost weight, you now have a larger percentage of body fat. In other words, you are actually fatter than when you began the diet.

Losing muscle tissue is a major health concern because muscle is the body-building tissue—the very tissue that burns calories most efficiently. Once you have shifted your percentage of lean to fat tissue, you'll find it even harder than before to lose weight because fat tissue requires fewer calories to sustain itself than muscle does. A reduction in muscle tissue is one reason dieters gain all the weight back and more as soon as they resume their previous eating habits. According to the *Harvard Heart Letter,* "typically as much as two-thirds of the lost weight is regained within one year, and almost all is regained within five years." This sets up a chronic dieter for the "yo-yo phenomenon."

Weight loss yo-yoing occurs when a large and rapid loss of weight is followed by an at least equally large and rapid gain in weight as soon as the dieter relaxes control. This occurs mainly because, in addition to a shift in lean-to-fat tissue, many people who achieve considerable weight loss experience, like their prehistoric ancestors, a reduction in their metabolic rates, and therefore a reduction in energy requirements, in their body's instinctual effort to defend against starvation. This allows the lost weight to be regained in a much shorter time than it was lost and means that the next time the person goes on a diet, losing the same amount of weight will take longer. In addition to frustrating the dieter, recent studies indicate that "weight cycling" may actually be more dangerous than maintaining a steady but slightly increased weight over time. Yo-yoing has been shown to damage health in several ways, including increasing the chances of heart disease and heart attacks, gout, osteoarthritis, diabetes, certain cancers, and other disorders.

Problems with Popular Diets

Millions of people who desperately want to lose weight find hope through the ever-present variety of diets. A few favorites, including low-fat and high-protein diets, recycle on a regular basis. These weight-loss notions fall into a whirlpool of increasingly contradictory information supplied by a number of reputable scientists.

While one specialist will tout a low-fat diet as the key to weight loss, another will say that the answer is not eating less fat. As proof, the proponent may point to the fact that for the past several years many of us have been eating less fat, yet we're still fatter than ever. Some surveys show that the proportion of calories Americans get from fat has dropped about 8 percent to 34 percent of our diet since the 1980s. Yet the prevalence of obesity has risen during the same time frame.

A diet high in carbohydrates was the rage throughout the 1980s and into the early 1990s. This rage was fueled by athletes' eating patterns, such as the popular "carbo-loading" the day before an event such as a marathon run. But recently people have been forced to take a second look at the beloved high-carbohydrate diets. These highly touted carbohydrates turned out to be sugars and starches, simple carbohydrates from processed foods, as distinguished from healthy complex carbohydrates. Now current research indicates that simple carbohydrates have a similar effect as fat—excesses are just as likely to be stored as fat as is fat itself. Plus, consuming high amounts of simple carbohydrates can cause the body to produce more insulin, which causes blood sugar to drop, which stimulates appetite.

Compounding the problem of high-carbohydrate diets is the fact that about 20 to 25 percent of the population is insulin-resistant. Insulin resistance impacts the body's ability to process carbohydrates properly, turning the sugars into fat and sending out an insistent demand for more carbohydrates. Insulin resistance is the result of constant increased demand for more insulin production by the pancreas, resulting in the production of poor-quality insulin that is not capable of effectively transferring glucose into muscle cells. When the muscle cell cannot receive the glucose, the body stores it as fat rather than allow the blood sugar to remain dangerously elevated. The high blood levels of insulin results in the rapid storage of fat since the body interprets the elevated insulin levels as abundant glucose immediately available for energy. Interestingly, the same insulin that was ineffective at getting glucose into the muscle cell is seemingly quite efficient at driving fat into the fat cells.

High-protein diets, the rage in the mid-1970s, are back again in the 1990s. This time they pit themselves against the high-carbohydrate and low-fat diets. These high-protein proponents point out that protein is essential for replacing and maintaining muscle. The more muscle you have, the higher your metabolism and the more calories you'll burn, even when you're not exercising. Also, eating more protein can help you feel fuller longer, since protein takes longer to digest and be absorbed than carbohydrates do. As a result, dieters will be less likely to nibble between meals or crave certain foods, which can reduce the overall number of calories you consume.

No matter how convincing the diet proponents are, the fact is that millions of people have tried these diets and are still fat. So no matter how rational the explanation of why a particular weight-loss diet is *the* diet to follow, not one as yet has the success numbers to back up its claims. If anything, we should have learned by now that no one diet works for everyone. And until each person's individual biochemistry and food intolerance is taken into consideration, the battle to reduce America's bulk will continue raging.

Side Effects of Diet Drugs

So if low-calorie, low-fat, and high-protein diets don't work, then diet drugs must be the answer to our weighty woes, right? Again, we're looking for the magic bullet, the effortless weight-loss approach that doesn't require us to become active participants in the acquisition and maintenance of our good health. So far the magic drug that lets us lose weight and continue our lives without lifestyle and dietary changes does not exist. Overweight is a sign that our lifestyles and food choices are inappropriate for our individual body chemistry. Overweight is beyond the scope of a "morning-after pill." Weight loss must become a personal crusade in which drugs serve only to temporarily distract us from hunger.

Many diet drugs used to treat severely obese people carry a heavy toll of side effects. For example, appetite suppressants help subside appetite but also stimulate the nervous system. Most drugs of this class are chemically related to amphetamines and may cause similar side effects. When such side effects appear, they are hardly conducive to long-term use of the drug. But when the drug is discontinued, the appetite returns with a vengeance, again pointing out our need to discover the underlying cause rather than focus on the symptoms of overweight.

Over-the-counter diet drugs may contain phenylpropanolamine, which can cause nausea, headaches, nervousness, elevated blood sugar levels, insomnia, and rapid heartbeat. Because these drugs are obviously not innocuous, we must treat them with care. According to Steven B. Karch in *The Pathology of Drug Abuse,* second edition, patients have experienced chest pain, arrhythmia, arrhythmic sudden death, seizures, and psychotic episodes. Stroke has also been reported with some frequency.

Over-the-counter diet-aid manufacturers are notorious for throwing in a little of everything legal to convince you that all the bases are covered. Formulations may include ginseng, licorice, ephedra, caffeine, and chromium, to name a few. Such ingredients are used for their chemical or drug-like effects and should be respected as such. Unfortunately, combining these concentrated drugs may compound the likelihood of serious side effects. For that reason, it's important that you know all the drugs you introduce to your body and their potential risks. Another serious drawback of diet drugs is that while they may help you lose weight by suppressing your appetite, your weight loss is usually temporary because the root cause of the overeating problem remains.

Current breakthroughs in the area of diet drugs involve those that increase the release of serotonin (the brain chemical that affects our mood and appetite). Fenfluramine (no longer available) stimulates the brain to release more serotonin, a neurotransmitter associated with pleasure and pain. Serotonin has been shown to influence appetite, helping people feel full and satisfied faster, thereby reducing calorie consumption and excess body weight in obese patients. Michael Weintraub, a clinical pharmacologist, made headlines in mid-1994 when news spread of his success in mixing fenfluramine with phentermine, a central nervous system stimulant. The combination of the "downer" and the "upper" was said to alter chemicals in the brain, producing a sense of balance and well-being. "Fen-phen" was touted as *the* magic solution to the battle of the bulge. It was said to go right to the heart of the problem for most dieters: "emotional" overeating, which is the hardest thing of all to overcome. But almost as quickly as it became the latest dieters' hope, fen-phen fell into the ranks of "dangerous" diet drugs.

As reported in a February 1995 ABC News *20/20* broadcast, researchers at Johns Hopkins University revealed the alarming fact that too high a dose of the mood-altering drug fenfluramine can produce brain damage, causing memory loss, anxiety, and nerve fiber destruction. A series of studies on laboratory animals showed that fenfluramine permanently destroys the very nerve fibers that produce the brain chemical serotonin. Some neurologists feared that this same effect could occur in humans as well. As a result, scientists warn that the safe range for human dosage is unknown and may be very narrow. Further, a May 1996 ABC News *PrimeTime Live* broadcast revealed a link between dexfenfluramine, also called Redux, and incurable lung disease. Specifically, 78 women developed primary pulmonary hypertension, which has an average survival rate of three years because high blood pressure in the lungs puts so much stress on the heart that it ultimately fails.

Further, the safety and effectiveness of FDA-approved Redux (no longer available) was not studied beyond one year. Although they've been highly touted by weight-loss clinics, most experts are recommending these diet drugs only for severely obese people, for whom the risks of carrying excess weight far outweigh the possible hazards. But even this thinking may be suspect because some research already shows that people taking fen-phen, like those taking other diet drugs, frequently return to former eating habits once they stop taking the drug. A four-year study on dexfenfluramine usage shows that nearly all who took the drug eventually regained their weight once they stopped the drug. In addition to the cost to our health, these diet drugs are not cheap. A year's supply costs an estimated $1,500. Fenfluramine (pondimin) and dexfenfluramine (redux) have been voluntarily removed from the market pending investigation of their possible role in the development of heart-valve damage.

The newest diet drug released to pacify the clamoring American public is Sibutramine. This latest testament to our national "state of denial" breezed through FDA approval in record time. Initial evaluation of the drug revealed that it was too dangerous and further study was necessary. Despite the recommendations of its own committee, the FDA approved Sibutramine for treatment of overweight. It is now available in pharmacies. The primary concerns with this drug are its tendency to elevate pulse and blood pressure and its short period of evaluation. Currently it is the only serotonergic drug approved for weight loss. It affects serotonin by inhibiting re-uptake. That is, it delays the normal reabsorption of serotonin by nerve cells, thus prolonging its hunger-suppressant effect. It too has significant risks and side effects, the most striking of which seems to be its propensity to elevate blood pressure in some patients to potentially dangerous levels. It is not clear whether Sibutramine may cause primary pulmonary hypertension, a rare but often fatal lung condition associated with some serotonergic drugs.

The "fat blocker" Orlistat was scheduled to be unleashed on the public this year but as yet it has not been released. Apparently problems appeared in early studies that the FDA could not overlook. Preliminary information on Orlistat reveals that one bothersome side effect may be leakage of fat-laden bowel contents. Researchers also question the effect of Orlistat on the absorption of fat-soluble vitamins. The human body has a carefully balanced physiology, and the arbitrary restriction of fat may interfere with many vital body functions.

It is evident that no perfectly safe drugs are on the horizon for the control of appetite or weight. Each patient must evaluate the potential benefits and risks and make his or her choice. One thing is clear: Unless a drug is used to cure a disease, it is only a stopgap. Ultimately some effort must be made to determine the underlying cause of a patient's overweight and a curative treatment instituted to turn the risk/benefit ratio in favor of the patient. For patients whose excess weight is due to food intolerance, appetite suppressants need be used only temporarily to assist them in the speedy elimination of their culprit foods.

"Feel Good" Foods

Current thinking concerning food intolerance and obesity is that reactive foods trigger or inhibit the brain chemicals such as serotonin that control appetite and food cravings. When these potent chemicals are thrown out of balance in our bodies, we uncontrollably crave foods, especially starchy and sugary foods that will give us a quick surge of serotonin. These foods have a "serotonergic" impact on the brain chemicals; in other words, they trigger the same calming "feel good" effect as the serotonergic drugs. Because this is a short-term effect, within an hour or two we need another food "fix." In a sense, we are medicating ourselves with food.

Research shows that when intolerant foods are eliminated from our diet, the effect is similar to that of mood-altering drugs, only infinitely healthier—the brain chemistry returns to normal and the compulsive food cravings disappear. Researchers have not yet identified exactly why this occurs, but know that an important relationship exists between the allergic response of the white blood cells and platelets to brain chemistry. So, it stands to reason that any disruption of the blood cells caused by allergenic foods could adversely impact the brain chemistry. With this safe, economical path to weight loss available to those with food intolerance, any rationale for the long-term use of drugs goes by the wayside.

While hard evidence to prove this theory may be a few years away, medical practitioners do know that when patients remove intolerant foods from their diets, food cravings go away. They lose excess fat—and lose it naturally, without the expense and side effects of powerful weight-loss drugs. Therefore, losing and keeping weight off begins by first identifying the individual's problem foods.

Modern Advances in Weight Loss

Currently, there is much hope and speculation in the medical world regarding genetic engineering. Using powerful new tools in molecular biology and genetic engineering, scientists in laboratories around the world are looking for cures for all kinds of disease, including obesity. Scientific theory regarding obesity says that we maintain our weight when our various metabolic feedback loops, tuned by whatever susceptibility genes we carry, settle into a happy equilibrium with our environment. The twentieth-century effects of the economic, cultural, and lifestyle changes are propelling more of us—in particular, those with more genetic risk factors—into obesity. But genetic-engineering researchers hope to someday find the hormone that will regulate metabolism and weight by, for example, signaling the brain that the body has stored enough fat.

Our understanding of how the body controls weight, or fails to do so, has began to develop in the 1950s. It has gained momentum since late 1994, when proponents of the genetic solution to obesity made many interesting and groundbreaking discoveries related to genes and obesity. Among the breakthroughs was the cloning of a mouse gene that has a role in telling the body to plump up or slim down. The gene is called Ob, for obese, because obesity is the result when the gene does not work properly in mice. Abnormalities in the genes can result in an abnormal protein that interferes with the body's complicated and delicate balance of biochemical pathways controlling appetite and the processing of food.

The following year scientists identified the gene's protein associated with eating behavior and metabolic rate and called it *leptin* (after the Greek word for thin). Studies have shown that leptin apparently helps determine how much fat a mouse is carrying. If there's too much, leptin tempers the appetite and speeds up metabolism to burn more calories. Scientists gave mice daily injections of leptin and, in just two weeks, the mice lost 30 percent of their body weight. However, by early 1996, before the dust surrounding this latest "breakthrough" had settled, *The New England Journal of Medicine* was reporting that, although it helped obese mice become thin, leptin didn't work the same way in humans. In fact, obese men and women appear to have plenty of leptin (four times more than people of normal weight), but they are unable to process its signal properly.

A follow-up study with human subjects showed that as food intake dropped, leptin levels dropped even further. The body's reaction to a decrease in food intake is to limit leptin's "stop-eating" signal. This could be one reason why rapid weight-loss programs don't work.

The early stage of genetic engineering has many drawbacks. The arena is so complex that scientists rarely find only one gene responsible for the problem in every person. Any single physiologic function is controlled by the interplay of several genes. For example, scientists have already located five genes that can cause rodents to gain weight. The best guess at this point is that obesity in humans is a polygenic disease, involving a number of genes that interact with each other and affect the biochemical pathways, which in turn influence our eating, metabolism, and physical activity. And that is only the beginning of the problem. Once they discover the genes, scientists must then determine just how each exerts its power on our bodies. Then treatments have to be proven safe in animals, and finally in humans. Clinical trials must also show whether the gene is effective in people whose fatness is often due to reasons other than just genetics.

What's more, while to some degree genetics are clearly involved in obesity, they cannot be the whole story. Proof is apparent when we look at specific populations of people who have been taken out of their traditional environment. The Pima Indians, for example, are commonly cited by experts. Despite a common genetic background between the Pima Indians in Arizona and those who live in Mexico, American Pimas have a far higher incidence of obesity—in part because many eat high-fat foods, whereas Mexican Pimas subsist mainly on grains and vegetables. The American Pimas lead a more sedentary lifestyle, while their Mexican cousins still actively engage in growing their own food and livestock and exhibit normal weight patterns. In a study of fat-storing genes and their impact on society, conducted by Eric Ravussin, Ph.D., and Clifford Bogardus, M.D., obesity researchers working for the National Institutes of Health in Arizona found more than 80 percent of the Arizona Indians weighed twice the national average. Most suffered from a host of medical conditions such as diabetes and gallbladder disease.

So the reengineering of a defective gene to make someone revert from fat to slender remains in the realm of theory and does not yet provide a practical solution. Considering all the challenges genetic researchers face, we can safely say that, despite encouraging advances, scientists are unlikely to discover miracle cures for the many chronic diseases that plague modern man. Once again, effective treatment boils down to each individual—finding which foods we must avoid, making sensible lifestyle modifications, and starting a practical exercise program.

The Biochemical Connection to Obesity

Ever wonder why you have an uncontrollable craving for a particular food even though you may not be truly hungry? For decades, medical practitioners have blamed overeating and obesity on a lack of willpower, a lack of discipline, poor self-control, or psychological problems resulting from an addictive personality or traumatic childhood experiences. Obese people have been viewed as psychologically flawed, driven to overeat by neurotic self-defeating urges. Those issues may indeed be part of the obesity problem in some people, but practitioners in the fields of psychology and medicine agree that such explanations are not valid for the entire one-half of the adult population who are overweight. Virtually no scientific evidence supports these explanations or suggests that people who struggle with weight are any different psychologically from those who do not. In spite of the absence of data, this stereotype persists among the public as well as within the medical community.

Many researchers in this area are convinced that obesity isn't a failure of will, but a chronic medical condition with complex biomedical roots. According to the *Harvard Medical School Harvard Heart Letter* (March 1994), "Medical researchers and weight-loss experts no longer regard being overweight as a simple failure of willpower. Instead, obesity is increasingly considered a chronic disease, like hypertension or diabetes." The fact is that almost 50 million Americans are dieting right now and, statistically, 95 percent of them will fail—so logically, there has to be another reason why people are too fat and why they can't lose and keep off weight.

Recent advances in research have opened a new chapter in our understanding of obesity. Now new and promising research points to the effects of our powerful brain chemicals on our ability to lose and our propensity to gain weight. After almost 20 years of research on the relationship between brain chemistry and eating behaviors, Dr. Sara Leibowitz, a neuroscientist at Rockefeller University, found that disturbances in eating behavior reflect disturbances in brain chemistry. What we eat, when we eat, and how much we eat is determined by the type of brain chemistry we have, not the type of personality. These findings may at last lead to better ways to stop the powerful forces within our body from working against our best efforts to shed unwanted pounds of fat. The search is on for ways to correct these biochemical abnormalities.

To understand the complex biochemical forces that control our actions, we can benefit from knowing something about our brain chemistry. To start with, real hunger signals come from an area of the brain called the hypothalamus, which controls the balance between the body's need for food and its use of energy. The hypothalamus is the brain's nerve-control center for many metabolic functions crucial to appetite control. It sends out powerful chemical messengers, called neurotransmitters and hormones, which influence when we eat, how much we eat, and what we eat. The ideal way for us to approach our diet is to eat only when our appetite is stimulated by hunger and to stop eating when the appetite is inhibited at the appropriate point by the sensation of satiety. Recent research indicates that integrating our internal and external stimuli to achieve this depends on our chemical and physiological makeup. Normally chemicals in our brain signal whether we are hungry or full. A defect in our system could lead to our overeating.

Our brain is the controller of food intake, receiving signals and sending signals, and adjusting the balance between metabolism and storage. We each have a number of specific neurotransmitters that are known to be involved in the integration and control of hunger and satiety, including gamma-aminobutyric acid (GABA), norepinephrine (noradrenaline), serotonin, dopamine, and histamine. Also, several neuropeptides (regulatory peptides able to affect the nervous system) are known to be involved, including neuropeptide Y, ß-endorphin, dynophine, growth hormone-releasing hormone, and galanin. All of these stimulate food intake when injected into special regions of the hypothalamus. For example, if you skip a meal or eat a very low-calorie diet, galanin sends one very persistent message: Eat and store fat. When we eat certain carbohydrates, levels of serotonin increase and we feel better. When operating at optimum levels, our body will naturally keep serotonin levels high and block galanin overproduction.

Other important players in obesity include hormones. Brain-made hormones called endorphins and amino acids (the building blocks of proteins) both act directly on the hypothalamus. Scientists have shown in animal experiments that high brain endorphin levels affect the craving for fatty foods. Obese animals were found to have higher levels of endorphins in their hypothalamus and larger appetites. The hormone insulin controls blood-sugar levels and signals the brain that the body has been fed. After a meal, insulin surges into the bloodstream, ordering our cells to suck up glucose and store it, and to absorb amino acids needed to build muscles and other tissues.

When insulin metabolism goes awry, as it can when you eat a food to which you are intolerant, levels of fats in the blood also go awry and you crave simple sugars. When you eat too much sugar and carbohydrates, the body releases insulin to bring down your blood-sugar levels into the normal range. One way this occurs is by pushing sugar out of the bloodstream and depositing it as fat. This system served our prehistoric ancestors well because it helped to ensure that they had the necessary fat reserves to make it through the next famine; however, this highly individualized insulin system is working against modern man's ability to maintain an ideal body weight.

Serotonin and the ALCAT Test

This chapter offers a brief glimpse of what's involved in the complex area of obesity and biochemistry. The exact roles of the many neurotransmitters and hormones involved in obesity are not yet clear and require further research. But based on current theories and preliminary research, we can make an educated guess that the effect of food intolerance on these powerful biochemical and genetic forces is significant. Take serotonin, for example, which controls how we feel: If we eat certain carbohydrates, serotonin levels increase and we feel better. Serotonin is a chemical substance primarily present in the white blood cells and platelets—the very cells that change due to the presence of allergenic foods. This change is what the ALCAT Test measures.

Research already conducted on the ALCAT Test shows that people who remove their food intolerances find that, among other things, their "cravings for sweets" is diminished.

This strongly suggests that food intolerances somehow impact serotonin functioning. In fact, one study on food allergy mediators conducted in Australia shows that eating an allergenic food often makes the blood levels of serotonin decline. Lower levels of serotonin make you uncomfortable, and you turn to simple sugars and carbohydrates for relief. Highly refined carbohydrates and sugars will cause a rapid release of insulin, which in turn reduces concentrations of all amino acids in the blood, except for tryptophan, a precursor of serotonin. Thus, in order to compensate for lower brain levels of serotonin, caused by eating the offending foods, food-sensitive people tend to crave foods that increase serotonin in the brain. This sets up a vicious cycle of food cravings and addiction. Medical science would bring in a drug at this point to temporarily relieve this craving; but research on food intolerance shows that you can get a permanent, non-pharmaceutical effect by removing the allergenic foods that trigger the serotonin imbalance in the first place.

ALCAT: The Bottom Line

Research already conducted on the ALCAT Test shows that people who remove their food intolerances find that, among other things, their "cravings for sweets" is diminished. This strongly suggests that the intolerant foods, which damaged the white blood cells, also disrupted the chemicals in those cells, thus continuing the patient's cycles of obesity and poor health.

The bottom line is that all the drawbacks of conventional weight-loss diets are removed when people follow diets that remove food intolerances as identified by the ALCAT Test. In the next few chapters, we'll explore the connection between weight loss and food intolerance, and illustrate how the ALCAT Test helps people identify their food intolerances and find their way back to their ideal weight.

CHAPTER 3

Breakthrough Research on Obesity and Health

At current rates, every single person in the United States will be obese by the year 2230.

> —from research cited by World Health Organization (WHO) task force, May 1996

The number of Americans with diabetes has jumped nearly 50 percent since 1983 and tripled since the late 1950s.

> —from a 1995 study by the National Institute of Diabetes

Twelve million Americans have asthma, and 5,000 die every year. Mortality has doubled since 1978.

> —Dr. Daniel M. Libby, clinical associate professor of medicine, Cornell University Medical College

More and more, doctors are seeing children with ear infections that don't respond to first-line treatments like amoxicillin, a type of penicillin.

> —*Austin American–Statesman,* July 12, 1996

The four statistics given opposite are just some of the many alarming reports on the state of our health as we exit the twentieth century. These statistics should surprise anyone familiar with the amazing advances that have taken place in the field of medicine in the twentieth century. One hundred years ago doctors could do little more than set broken bones, lance boils, and soothe symptoms; they could seldom cure disease. All that changed by the middle of the century. Medical science began making breathtaking advances and medicine began triumphing over many health problems such as infectious diseases, heart disease, some cancers, brain disease, and immune system malfunctions, to name a few.

And yet, as we exit this amazing century in medicine and enter the twenty-first century, medical science is still battling some common illnesses that cripple and kill millions of people around the world. Not only are we seemingly losing ground on some health problems that have been around for decades, but we're also facing a growing number of new problems.

This predicament forces the question—what exactly is going on? The United States has the greatest medical science in the world, yet a good deal of today's research points to one shocking fact—as a whole, we're getting fatter and sicker. Clearly, part of the medical puzzle is still missing—and that missing piece is keeping too many of us and our children from the optimal health we all desire. This situation does not result from a lack of effort to find solutions; it may instead result from looking for answers in the wrong places or looking at our health from the wrong perspective.

Medical science has no shortage of new treatments and new research underway for ever-new understanding of the human body, the nature of specific diseases, and cures for those diseases. Every day, in popular magazines, daily newspapers, and television and radio reports, we hear about the latest medical treatments and research.

For example, obesity has recently been cited as the second biggest health concern of our age. Indeed, this is no small health problem: Obesity alone accounts for the overwhelming increase in diabetes, heart disease, and high blood pressure. An immense amount of ground-breaking research is currently underway in the worldwide effort to find a solution to this nearly out-of-control medical problem. Today drug therapy, gene manipulation, hormonal activity, and other biochemical functions are currently under intense scrutiny in laboratories around the world—researchers are conducting hundreds of studies in their search for a way to end what's been called "the plague of our age."

New Hope for the Overweight

All this research on obesity sounds exciting and full of potential, but within the mountains of study conclusions, few offer definitive solutions. The prognosis for a life of ideal weight is still grim into the foreseeable future.

In the middle of this storm of speculation and disappointment, one obesity and health research study was quietly conducted in 1995 at Columbia/HCA Medical Center's Sports Medicine and Performance Center in Houston and at Baylor Medical College. One hundred overweight patients who had at least two other health problems, such as migraines and chronic tiredness, were studied. This four-week trial, which studied the impact of food intolerance on obesity and other common health problems, led to extraordinary results.

The 50 study participants who eliminated foods identified by a simple blood test measuring adverse reactions in their bodies lost not just body weight but body fat. In fact, these subjects lost an average of nearly three pounds of fat and gained almost one pound of lean muscle. The 50 "control" subjects, on the other hand, who followed their own weight-loss plans, gained an average of one pound of fat and lost almost one pound of lean muscle. Overall, the two groups' body composition (lean-to-fat ratio) showed a six-pound difference at the end of the four-week trial. Calculated from a statistical perspective, these differences are highly significant.

Still more astounding, the participants in the experimental group improved significantly and dramatically in 20 of 24 disease symptoms when compared to their counterparts who followed dietary plans of their own choosing. This study achieved results—measurable changes in body weight, body composition, and disease symptoms with a simple, non-pharmaceutical therapy. "We found that you can change people's health dramatically when you remove their intolerant foods from their diets," noted the principal investigator of the study, Dr. Gilbert Kaats, Ph.D. Dr. Kaats, who is the director of the Health and Medical Research Foundation, an independent research organization in San Antonio, added that "[determining] food intolerance is extremely helpful in improving health and losing weight. It's much more effective than traditional dieting."

Common Foods Can Sabotage Your Health

Dr. Kaats's breakthrough study demonstrated a remarkable and unprecedented occurrence within the bodies of the 50 "experimenters" (as they're called in research parlance) who eliminated the respective foods to which each was shown to be biochemically sensitive. What occurred? By not eating their intolerant foods, the 50 "experimenters" eliminated substances that disrupted their body's immune system, brain chemistry, and/or digestive system.

These findings are among the first to support a theory that a growing number of medical doctors have held for decades: By eliminating "intolerant" foods from a person's diet, you remove the substances that trigger the health problems in the first place. Thse foods have been exacerbating the problems through repeated exposure.

The United States has the greatest medical science in the world, yet a good deal of today's research points to one shocking fact—as a whole, we're getting fatter and sicker.

For example, the immune system may have overreacted to what it perceived as an "invader" (the intolerant food or a chemical in the food), which it then attacked, just as it would attack a virus or a bacteria. Or the intolerant foods may have caused the body's sensitive brain chemistry to go haywire, creating food cravings that triggered eating binges or disrupted metabolism; or they compounded digestive system deficiencies, resulting in malabsorption that exacerbated the obesity and health problems. Once one or more of these reactions begins, the body's systems are no longer able to operate at optimum performance.

Once their troublemaking foods were out of the way, the research participants' immune systems, brain chemistry, and digestive systems were no longer struggling to operate under adverse conditions. Instead, they adjusted to the healthier internal "climate" and functioned at maximum performance—metabolizing the safe foods more effectively, burning stored fat more efficiently, neutralizing food cravings, eliminating water retention, and clearing away health symptoms. "Our findings are consistent with the latest biochemical and genetic research," Dr. Kaats adds. "It looks like when some people eat certain foods, which could be anything from milk products to lettuce, they experience an allergic-like reaction. With regards to weight loss, instead of getting a rash or going into anaphylactic shock, their appetite and food cravings increase. Eliminating these allergenic foods appears to balance appetite, food cravings, and body composition."

The World That Technology Built

Exactly what do the current statistics on the state of our health at the turn of this century say about our sophisticated medical technology? And what do the results of this small research study, which took such a simple step to correct health problems and got such dramatic results, say about treating today's mounting health-care problems? You can find answers to these questions by looking back 100 years ago, to before medical science and medical technology transformed the world by creating cures and treatments for many of the ills of the human body. As medical science began to take off in the early 1900s, it naturally focused on the health-care epidemics of the time—tuberculosis, bacterial infections, scarlet fever, and smallpox, to name a few. By mid-century, as research moved us toward greater technological advances in heart, brain, and cancer treatments, for example, it took a definitive turn that shaped the "traditional" medical treatment we receive today, including the development of potent pharmaceuticals.

In the race to find treatments and cures for the ailments of the nineteenth century, medical science appears to have had one major shortcoming—it could not keep up with the problems that were developing, ironically, as a result of twentieth-century technology. (In all fairness, nobody had a crystal ball that allowed him or her to peer into the future and see what troubles were brewing.) The outcome was that researchers and doctors, by and large, were not able to address the "new" health problems. These problems were being created and compounded by the very developments in medical science that were supposed to eradicate health problems in our lifetimes. Technological developments in other industries further exacerbated the health threat to twentieth-century Americans. As it was, medical science was not the only industry making giant leaps forward in technology.

With the twentieth century nearly behind us, we can look back and see clearly how our world changed in a hundred years. For example, while our forefathers traveled by horse and buggy, we travel by car, train, and plane. While a century ago all farming was "organic," today each of us consumes pounds of chemicals each year, all added as we grow, transport, package, and cook our food. And while people at the turn of the twentieth century lived slow-paced lives close to home, today we travel daily to offices miles from home, sit in rush-hour traffic, and largely communicate with each other by such impersonal modes as phone, fax, and e-mail. No one would argue that in 100 years we've created a very different world.

The net result of such changes is that while doctors around the world advanced from mere lancing of boils and setting of bones to performing incredible medical miracles, our world was becoming increasingly adulterated. The amazing technological advances that have changed our planet more in the last 100 years than in the entire previous history of the human race, have also brought a slew of environmental health hazards in the form of air pollution, water pollution, and heavily adulterated and nutritionally deficient foods. In the final analysis, this downside to progress may well be the core of many, if not all, of today's mounting health-care problems. Ironically, as technology has become more sophisticated, aimed toward making our lives better, it has placed our bodies in a relatively unnatural existence—both internally and externally.

A High-Tech Solution to Health Care

Clearly, we now need health care that takes into account the world that twentieth-century technology has created. We must find the missing puzzle piece that will stop diseases like obesity, diabetes, asthma, ear infections, attention deficit disorder, and other health problems from running rampant. This elusive piece may not be a miracle drug or expensive surgical procedure; it may be as simple as removing the foods that contribute to the twentieth-century overload with which our bodies contend daily.

Luckily, along with other high-tech developments in medical science, a simple test has been invented that easily and quickly analyzes blood cells to determine the exact foods, food chemicals, and other substances to which a person is intolerant. Although many medical practitioners (called "environmental physicians") used the food intolerance concept to treat patients in previous decades, they could only help a limited number of people because testing was a slow, tedious, often uncomfortable process.

This research on health and obesity and other studies on food intolerance using the new blood-testing procedure have led researchers to discover that the simple step of removing intolerant foods brings permanent relief from often chronic health-care problems that no medicine or procedure previously could resolve. Others have benefitted from overall changes in how they live their lives and treat their bodies. To make significant strides in medicine in the coming century, we need to address the real world of chemicals, pollution, and modern stressors. And to effectively do that, we must add food intolerance testing to the physician's bag of great medical treatments available today.

Food Intolerance:
Breakthrough Diagnosis and Treatment

Have you ever gone to a doctor and complained of a headache, tiredness, an upset stomach, or some other persistent condition? If so, what did the doctor say? "Take two aspirin" or "Get more sleep." Maybe they did some test then said, "Nothing's wrong, it must all be in your head." Or quite possibly they simply gave you a prescription for some drug. If you or someone you know has experienced such medical treatment, you're not alone. Thousands of people receive this diagnosis every day in medical offices across America. Is it any wonder that most people do not share such chronic, low-grade symptoms with their physicians?

What about the last weight-loss diet you went on? Did it leave you feeling hungry, low on energy, cranky and nervous, or craving particular foods like sweets? Then, after all the trouble of counting calories, cutting back on fats, and feeling awful, did you finally give in, binge on the foods you craved, and gain back the weight you lost? This is the sad story for millions of dieters across the country every day. They eat salads, drink skim milk, and sip bottled water, at least until they can't take it anymore and devour a donut or consume a bag of chips in 30 seconds flat. Then they start thinking about how they can get their hands on the next food they crave. This is a troubling, stressful life for our powerful, yet delicate bodies. It's no wonder that as a nation we're fatter than ever.

Or perhaps you're the parent of a child with chronic ear infections, or one who's been labeled with hyperactivity/attention deficit disorder (ADHD). Maybe your child's chronic headaches and stomachaches cost you precious hours visiting the doctor's office, taking time off from work, or lying awake at night? Do doctors recommend surgery to insert ear tubes or prescription drugs like Ritalin to deal with your child's health problems? If so, you have a lot of company. Today, there is a literal epidemic of children diagnosed with otitis media (ear infections) and ADHD—and the traditional medical treatments for these two conditions are surgery and drugs. What message do we give our children about their health care now and in the future?

The Modern World Confounds Traditional Medicine

If any of the above situations remind you of your experiences or those of someone you know, welcome to traditional twentieth-century medicine. It's a world of surgery and prescription drugs, and little else. And it's guided by an impersonal, efficient philosophy that focuses on treating the symptoms rather than the sources of health problems. Meanwhile, the modern world is full of stress, pollution, and preservative-filled, chemically packed, and genetically altered "food." And it appears certain that the next century will share the legacy. But do these factors play a part in the medicine doctors practice on our bodies? The sad answer is not often. One study, for example, found that less than four percent of the population gets their nutritional information from their doctors. Interestingly, the same study, conducted by the American Dietetic Association for its 1995 Nutritional Trends Survey, reported that 39 percent of the population say they get most of their nutritional information from magazines.

Meanwhile, medical companies give the illusion of accomplishing great things in these same magazines. You can hardly pick up a newspaper or magazine without reading an advertisement or article for another "breakthrough drug" to treat arthritis, depression, weight loss, asthma, or any of a long list of common medical problems. What's more, billions of dollars go into research to develop pharmaceuticals, therapies, and medical equipment to treat our ailments. We have access to all these phenomenal medical accomplishments, yet as a nation are sicker and fatter than ever. In fact, for all the trillions spent on medical care, we have seen surprisingly little progress in combating major and minor diseases.

Look at any illness—including diabetes, arthritis, asthma, cancer, and obesity—and you'll find that it's on the rise instead of the decline. Yet when you see advertisements for the latest drugs and therapies, you'd expect everyone to be brimming with health—all we have to do is take those magic pills. Something is wrong with this picture. Modern medicine focuses largely on treating symptoms, and all but ignores the sources of our mounting health ills.

More than one critic has expressed concern for the current state of our health-care system. For example, in his book *Dear America, A Concerned Doctor Wants You to Know the Truth about Health Reform,* published in 1993, Melvin Konner, M.D., wrote:

What has happened to American medicine's Golden Age? Just a couple of decades ago it seemed as though doctors could do no wrong. Medical miracles lay like jewels to be picked up each time we turned a corner. Penicillin, streptomycin, cortisone, polio vaccine, open-heart surgery, the heart-lung machine, psychiatric drugs, kidney dialysis, transplants—three decades ago there seemed to be no end to what we could do, and no limit to medicine's confidence. America clearly did have the best health care in the world, and it seemed sure only to get better. Yet today there is widespread agreement that the system is not working.

Our health care is now to the point that we have to ask ourselves: Are these expensive, high-tech therapies helping or are they hurting our health?

The Summer 1995 edition of *Health & Wellness Today*, published by Julian Whitaker, M.D., states:

- Doctors get free vacations, computers, cellular phones, even free educations for prescribing certain drugs— whether or not they are good for you!

- In a major study, Boston University researchers found that 36 percent of hospital admissions are caused by doctors' blunders!

- A seven-year study of 90,000 women, ages 40–59, showed that those who had regular mammograms were subjected to twice the surgical procedures and more mastectomies than those who didn't—yet life expectancy is exactly the same! Mastectomies were used for over 100 years before anyone did a study to see if they were effective (they weren't).

- Balloon angioplasty—a $4 billion-per-year business— kills 9,000 people a year . . . even though there's never been a study to prove it does any good! Heart bypass operations—a $10 million-per-day industry—kill 28,000 Americans every year, even though two big studies have proven bypass surgery does *not* make patients live longer!

- Even doctors admit that 900,000 unnecessary angiograms are done every year in the U.S. alone. And 4,500 people die needlessly as a result!

- Each year, two million patients pick up hospital infections that they didn't have before they were admitted. Of those, about 60,000 die from the infection.

And if the way doctors are practicing medicine today isn't working, what then is the way to achieve the optimum health that we all desire and deserve?

The Environmental Epidemic of the Twentieth Century

When, if ever, will our health-care system take into account the mounting adulterations our bodies have to deal with in today's world—pollution, stress, and food chemicals. Pollution has been a growing health problem for decades, has even been linked to death. An environmental advocacy group, the Natural Resources Defense Council, released a report in early 1996 linking certain types of air pollution—combustion of coal, oil, gas, diesel, and wood, and high-temperature processing such as copper smelting and steel mills—to the premature deaths of about 64,000 Americans a year. Stress has been a known detriment to poor health for decades—yet our society only encourages more and more stress-producing lifestyles. Then there is the problem of increasing chemicals and genetically engineered food. In fact, Drs. Miller and Ashford, in their book *Chemical Exposures,* allege that each year every adult consumes 24 pounds of man-made chemicals.

Given these challenging conditions—and they are just the tip of the iceberg—is it any wonder that food intolerance is growing more prevalent as many specialists suggest? Indeed, it may even be, as many predict, the epidemic of the late century. Estimates on the prevalence of food intolerance range from 30 percent to 90 percent of the population suffering from some degree of the condition. Perhaps food intolerance is a sign that the human body has not fully adapted to the novel environment we have created for ourselves. Is this the legacy we want to pass on to our children in the twenty-first century?

The Cost of Bad Health and Poor Health Care

Many are profiting from our ill health—drug companies, diet product companies, developers of expensive medical technologies, makers of convenience foods—and the list goes on. Everyone, it seems, is profiting but us. The American health-care system is among the biggest profit enterprises in the country. In 1992, according to the U.S. Commerce Department, Americans spent $847 billion on health care. By 1995, the cost of treating disease had reached in excess of $1 trillion. By the year 2000, health-care costs are expected to reach an astonishing $1.3 trillion. It's nearly impossible to determine the amount of money spent on any given disease; too many factors must be considered. But one thing is certain: it's costing more every year to treat any given disease. Take a look at just one of today's most common diseases: diabetes. Of the eight million Americans diagnosed with diabetes (it's believed that another eight million are undiagnosed), direct medical costs per year in the U.S. are $45 billion, while the indirect cost from disability is approaching another $47 billion, according to the National Institutes of Health.

Pharmaceutical companies, each of which has a large advertising budget, are among the most profitable corporations. They produce a large variety of increasingly more expensive drugs, and they profit however they can. Drug companies' attempts to further increase their profits through underhanded measures is the subject of many reports. One such report appeared in the *Wall Street Journal* on April 25, 1996. The article tells how one of the biggest drug companies paid a university to conduct a study on a new drug for hypothyroidism, a metabolic disorder that affects a diagnosed eight million Americans. Then the drug company undermined the results because the study found the new drug was virtually identical to three cheaper versions. The study also found that U.S. healthcare costs could be cut by $356 million a year if the new drugs were replaced by the cheaper, but equally effective, drugs. When one hears stories like this, it's easy to understand why people are often disillusioned with twentieth-century medicine.

Time for a New Medical Paradigm

What if medicine were practiced differently? What if the whole body were taken into consideration when a patient presented a chronic complaint? What if stress, pollution, and the foods we eat day in and day out were considered in our overall health? What if treatment of food intolerance were considered a viable route to good health? Surely, medicine would take a big turn for the better. It's difficult to precisely analyze the cost savings if a person were to prevent a disease from developing in the first place. But it's easy to imagine incredible savings if thousands of people did not acquire diabetes, arthritis, obesity, gastrointestinal problems, and a host of other common illnesses, thereby avoiding untold years of doctor visits, drug therapies, surgeries, and time off work.

Here's what a few of today's experts in food intolerance have to say about this therapy:

> The scientific investigations increasingly point toward the importance of applying food intolerance testing to patients'

overall health care. It's extremely important that practitioners put action behind their words, and do more to both prevent and treat this popular disease.

—Dr. Lene Høj, an internal medical doctor and specialist
in allergic diseases who operates a large private practice
in Copenhagen, Denmark

If food intolerance treatments were widely used, we'd see many more chronic conditions improve, including depression, mood swings, and overweight.

—Dr. John Magauran, a general practitioner
in private practice in Honolulu, Hawaii

I think that it's underestimated how many problems are related to food intolerance.

—Dr. Jay Sandweiss, an internal medicine practitioner
specializing in environmental medicine in Detroit

The possibility that diet may play a significant role in some patients and the usually benign nature of investigation required make it worthwhile to attempt to answer this question in any chronic disorder which is otherwise not adequately treatable or in which the usual prescribed treatment carries with it some hazard or adverse effect.

—Dr. Douglas H. Sandberg, the director of the Department
of Pediatrics, Division of Gastroenterology and Nutrition,
in the Allergic and Environmental Disease Unit at the
University of Miami Children's Hospital Center in Miami

I've had a great deal of satisfaction treating diet-related problems, for by doing so one gets to the root of the problem, and away from simply dishing out medications which treat symptoms, and provide only symptomatic relief.

—Dr. John Gerrard, an allergy and immunology specialist
and former Professor of Pediatrics at the
University of Saskatchewan in Saskatchewan, Canada

Most of the people I see have three common problems—
fatigue, depression, and difficulty with concentration, which
they don't even mention until after they've eliminated their
intolerant foods and those symptoms clear up. Many patients have told me, "I've had those symptoms for years and
now they're gone." That's nice to hear.

—Dr. Richard Bahr, an environmental medicine specialist
in private practice in Cincinnati

With any other traditional therapy you have side effects,
whereas with food intolerance testing there is no down side,
and there is an absolute up side.

—Dr. David Cafarelli, a medical practitioner specializing
in nutrition in West Palm Beach

Food Intolerance to the Rescue

It's time we actually did live our day-to-day lives with the
vim and vigor portrayed in magazine advertisements. It's
time we lived free from unnecessary chronic health complaints. And it's time we lived life to the fullest instead of
being needlessly weighted down by poor health and obesity. By addressing food intolerance, thousands of people
already made this goal a reality because they took a step
that is rarely mentioned in traditional medicine—they removed the *cause* of their health complaints, instead of
just masking the *symptoms* with a drug or other medical
treatment. Many have already found that the cure for
their health problems, whether minor or severe, was as
simple as removing foods that, for one reason or another,
did not agree with their systems.

If food intolerance is so widespread, why, you may
wonder, haven't you heard about it until now? That's a
good question. And the answer is firmly rooted in the fact
that food intolerance does not, for some reason, fit into
the modern, "traditional" model of medicine. Many doc-

tors simply do not accept it as a viable medical condition. The seed of this thinking begins in medical school, where the human body is broken into pieces to be studied and treated. As a result, if you have a sore throat you go to an ear, nose, and throat specialist; if you have a stomach problem you go to a gastroenterologist; and if you have a yeast infection you go to a gynecologist. This medical paradigm leaves little room for a treatment that requires a doctor to acknowledge that what a person puts in his or her mouth may cause a pain in his head, an infection in her ear, or itchy skin on his groin. Many doctors who practice what's called "alternative" medicine have broken out of the traditional mold and taken a different path—either because of a personal health experience or because they took a critical look at traditional medicine and didn't like what they saw.

For all the billions spent on medical care, we have seen surprisingly little progress in combating major and minor diseases.

Ironically, Hippocrates himself, the "Father of Medicine," said 2,500 years ago:

> It appears to me necessary to every physician to be skilled in
> nature, and to strive to know, if he would wish to perform
> his duties, what man is in relation to the articles of food and

drink, and to his occupations, and what are the effects of each of them to every one.

Yet today, as mentioned, food and nutrition are rarely discussed in the thousands of doctors' offices across the country.

Prescription Drugs: Just Say "No"?

Medical treatment typically consists of giving a chemical to relieve, cover up, or resolve a disease process, while the principal treatment of food intolerance consists of removing the offending agent. By disconnecting the parts of the body, medical practitioners disregard the impact one part of the body may have on another, which leads to another major aspect of medicine today—prescription drugs. If you're treating a disease as an entity, separate from all other functions of the body, then why not simply zap it with a drug? Never mind the short- and long-term side effects that drug may have on other organs of the body. Right now you're successful at relieving the migraine, infection, joint pain, ADHD, or weight problem.

Antibiotics alone, while powerful drugs that have saved many lives, also contribute to many health problems. Earlier this century, breakthroughs in antibiotics inspired confident predictions that all kinds of modern-day illnesses would be eradicated. But antibiotics have a sinister side—an adverse effect on the intestinal wall. The small intestine is host to not just unfriendly bacteria, but to the friendly bacteria that we need to keep our digestive system healthy. Antibiotics act like a Hoover, vacuuming out all bacteria, whether unfriendly or friendly. Due to an overuse of antibiotics since they were introduced in the 1930s, many of us are faced with the consequences—chronic illness.

Another factor facing modern health care is wave after wave of drug-resistant microbes: and we are running out of antibiotics to fight them. Just one example of this problem is illustrated in the preliminary findings of a two-year study on the use of antibiotics to treat chronic ear infections conducted at the University of Texas. The study found that more and more doctors were seeing children with ear infections who didn't respond to first-line antibiotic treatments (as many as 50 percent). This was forcing the doctors to resort to stronger drugs that cause diarrhea and upset stomachs. This problem has developed because bacteria have an incredible ability to become resistant to antibiotics.

Is the Cure Worse Than the Disease?

Despite the inconveniences, prescription drugs won't lose their luster any time soon. For one thing, drugs are a quick treatment. A doctor can write a prescription in 30 seconds, whereas discussing nutrition and other preventative health-care concerns could take hours. Clearly, by prescribing drugs, a physician can see more patients per day and have a more profitable practice. Of course, prescription drugs have their place in medicine; few medical practitioners would dispute that fact. But a growing number of medical practitioners and patient advocacy groups suspect that the prescription drug trend is getting out of control—to the detriment of the health it's designed to improve. On this note, John Braithwaite made an interesting observation in his book *Corporate Crime in the Pharmaceutical Industry*. He pointed out in a chapter entitled "The Corporation as Pusher" that "People who foster dependence on illicit drugs such as heroin are regarded as among the most unscrupulous pariahs (outcasts) of modern civilization. In contrast, pushers of licit (legal) drugs tend to be viewed as altruistically motivated purveyors of a social good. Yet dependence on Valium or Darvon can have consequences just as frightening as heroin addiction."

On this note, it's important to mention the perhaps most overused medication "pushed" on a frighteningly high number of our children—Ritalin. This amphetamine-like agent is standard therapy for hyperactive children, despite the fact that this drug is addictive and can cause psychotic behavior. In fact, Ritalin is one of the most popular forms of "speed" in the drug culture, drawing high prices in the illicit drug trafficking trade. Furthermore, Dr. Sidney Wolfe, head of a respected Washington public interest group that, among other things, evaluates drugs for consumers, pointed out in the early 1990s that 104 of the 287 most frequently prescribed drugs are too dangerous to use.

Prescription drugs are not the only medicines that may be undermining the health of many people. More than one study has found that over-the-counter medications may be more harmful that people realize. Case after case deals with people who took common pain relievers, asthma medications, cough and cold medicines, or nasal sprays and suffered joint pain, headaches, swollen blood vessels, indigestion, heartburn, liver damage, even death. Often doctors and the FDA blame the people themselves for using the medications incorrectly. But the fact is that most medication that has a good effect in one part of your body also has a negative side effect, usually on some other part of the body.

Aspirin, for example, one of the most common drugs used today, has a wide range of actions and a long list of beneficial effects, but also has one or two drawbacks. Every aspirin a person takes will slightly damage the intestinal wall and lead to a small amount of bleeding. The higher the dose, the greater the bleeding and damage. It's been found that a weakened gut wall, the only barrier between the body's digestion and elimination system and the bloodstream, can lead to severe health problems, including food intolerance. This is not the side effect a person needs when they take a small pill to get rid of a headache or joint pain. It's like taking one step forward and two steps back in our race to achieve long-term maximum health.

Walking the High Road to Wellness

Clearly, it's time we take a serious look at the way health care is practiced today so we can direct it down a more successful path tomorrow. And it's time we bring the successful, so-called "alternative" treatment of food intolerance out of the shadows and give many who suffer from poor health a chance to live free of disease. Consider this: Some medical practitioners estimate that 90 to 95 percent of all chronic illnesses are preventable. One of the easiest ways to keep people healthy is to avoid sickness or detect illness early.

But implementing this philosophy will require a paradigm shift in the thinking of our traditional medical practitioners, and in that of the insurance companies and HMOs that now control access to health care. Since HMOs profit by keeping sick people out of the system, this philosophy should fit in well with their business plans. By taking an active role in promoting good health, giving people access to the health-care services and tools, such as diagnostic tests, HMOs can ensure maximum health— clearly a win-win situation for both the companies and their patients.

CHAPTER 4

A Short Course in the Science of Food Intolerance

The body's immune system includes teams of specialized cells, some of which contain arsenals of powerful chemicals. These cells are like loyal and eager troops of foot soldiers, awaiting instructions from their commanding officers, prepared to defend the body from foreign invaders at a moment's notice. Armed with chemicals such as histamine, they are known as preformed mediators—typically inactive, but always awaiting the signal that will cause their release. Enter a non-friendly bacteria, virus, or parasite, and immune cells are brought to attention, prepared to release their chemical weapons to fight the invader.

The Role of the Immune System

The immune system must contend with numerous potential allergen types and has thus evolved a broad repertoire of responses to deal with the various situations it encounters. An outburst of chemicals is one of the many actions that keep us safe. Although the immune system comprises a sophisticated mechanism of self-defense, literally fighting enemies around the clock, occasionally a glitch occurs; for example, when the body develops an allergy to an otherwise harmless substance, such as a peanut or cat dander. Thus, the same powerful chemical response that is usually directed toward foreign pathogens, such as bacteria, viruses, and parasites, can react as powerfully against an innocuous substance, one that is harmless to most individuals. The immune response can even be directed against its own tissue, a sort of "friendly fire" phenomenon, causing an autoimmune disorder. The severity of reactions varies from mild and barely noticeable to life threatening, such as when a person goes into anaphylactic shock, causing serious illness and possibly death.

In 1906 an Austrian physician named von Pirquet coined the term "allergy" to mean "altered reaction." Thus any pathological response to a normally benign substance was referred to as an altered reaction, or allergy. However, a few decades later, allergists in Europe decided to narrow this definition to describe only such a reaction as occurs in rapid response to exposure to an allergen, such as the appearance of hives immediately following ingestion of shellfish or a sudden burst of sneezing following the inhalation of dust. The operative word here is "rapid." When such a reaction concerns a food, the very nature of the reaction, being immediate or very near immediate, makes identifying the culprit food quite easy. This contrasts with the bodys' reaction to delayed or hidden food allergies, usually referred to as sensitivities, in which symptom onset may take several hours to a couple of days to occur. Hence, delayed food allergies are much more difficult to diagnose; this is why they are called "hidden."

So, when a classical allergy reaction to a food occurs, identification is easy because the symptoms occur immediately after ingestion. However, immediate, or "classical," allergy reactions to airborne substances are difficult to identify because the air contains so many different things at any given time. Thus, diagnostic testing, using either skin response or blood testing, is appropriate for airborne allergens. These techniques, however, don't work for delayed reactions to foods or chemicals.

A brief history of the testing for both classical and hidden allergies is useful in order to understand why the latter has not received the recognition it is due. For decades, what caused these so-called classical or immediate allergy reactions was not known; however, allergists referred to the unknown agent as *reagin*. Then, in 1967, two independent teams of researchers, one from the Karolinska Institute in Sweden, and a husband and wife team in Colorado named Ishizaka, identified *reagin* as an IgE antibody. "Ig" in medical speak means "immunoglobulin." Immunoglobulin E (IgE) is the least common of the five major antibody types produced by the immune system. Through further investigation these researchers discovered how IgE (now understood to be the reaginic antibody) happens to cause the familiar symptoms of classical allergy—namely, increased mucus secretion and blood vessel permeability; smooth muscle constriction, inflammation, dilation of blood vessels, and stimulation of nerve endings; itching, general discomfort, and pain.

When a foreign protein enters the body, either through inhalation, direct contact with the skin, or ingestion, it may or may not make it through the initial defenses set up at the point of entry. If the foreign body does get past the barricade, a cell, such as a macrophage (meaning "big eater") or dendritic cell, will very likely take it up.

These will then break down the protein and transport the broken-down peptides on to the cell's own surface. The molecule that transports the allergen's peptides to the cell's surface is called a Major Histocompatibility II molecule, or MHC receptor for short. The macrophage or other cell performing this function, such as a dendritic cell, is called an *antigen-presenting cell*.

In the blood, lymph, and certain specialized tissue exists a type of white blood cell known as a *lymphocyte*. Different types of lymphocytes do different things. A T-helper II lymphocyte, or T cell for short, responds to the presentation of an allergen or antigen (antibody generator). ("T cells" get their name because they mature in the thymus, while "B cells" are so named because they mature in the bone marrow.) However, the T cell must have a receptor on its surface that conforms to the shape of the peptides of the allergen, and the MHC molecule presented to it.

If it does conform, and this is the basis of specific immunity, that T cell and only those T cells with the same receptor type will get switched on, that is, become activated. It then will bind with another type of lymphocyte known as a B lymphocyte if, and only if, the B cell also shares the same molecular structure, or receptor, on its surface. A chemical signal is then transmitted from the T cell to the B cell. The B cell gets switched on, transforms itself to a *plasma cell*, and begins to manufacture and then secrete soluble forms of that very same type of receptor into the blood. This soluble form of the receptor is an antibody, or immunoglobulin (globule of immunity). Remember, this type of receptor, or antibody, has a shape on one part that complements the original shape of the allergen components that started this whole sequence of events. Therefore, it will tend to bind with that allergen whenever the two come within close proximity. This is an important point.

As mentioned, those soluble receptors are called antibodies. If the intercellular signal sent from the T cell to the B cell involves a chemical called IL4, or Interleukin 4, the antibody that the B cell secretes is of the IgE type. What happens next is what the famous discoveries were all about. The IgE antibody, like other antibodies, has a "Y" shape to it. The stem portion of the "Y" has the propensity to bind with receptors on yet another type of white blood cell, a *mast cell*, or a similar type of cell known as a *basophil*. Mast cells are located in tissues, such as the lining of the gastrointestinal tract, the respiratory tract, the genitourinary tract, and the skin. Basophils, like mast cells, contain histamine, but they circulate in the blood.

Once bound to the mast cell or basophil, the portion of the IgE antibodies that remains unbound is the part that expresses the molecular configuration complementary to the shape of the peptides of the original allergen. Thus, it is known as an *allergen-specific antibody*. The next time that allergen comes around, it binds to the exposed portions of the allergen-specific IgE antibodies. When this happens, the mast cell or basophil reacts. The small granules within the cells, which contain histamine, are spewed out and cause the various allergy symptoms. The process, known as *degranulation*, happens quite quickly.

The immune system is believed to have evolved this particular response to defend against parasites, usually relatively large entities compared to white blood cells. Therefore this dramatic spewing of poisonous chemicals is necessary to effectively deter them. Why it occurs under inappropriate circumstances, such as a response to ragweed pollen, for instance, is unknown; but the tendency is inherited. On the positive side, people who tend to express this type of allergy, known as *atopy*, are in fact less susceptible to parasitic infections.

Following the initial distress caused by the release of preformed mediators (such as histamine, in this case), the immune system later converts the phospholipids, which make up the membranes of the involved cells, into other inflammatory mediator types. These mediators, known as *lipid mediators* and including prostaglandins and leuko-trienes, are responsible for the so-called *late phase reaction,* which takes place some six to eight hours later and lasts much longer than the initial reaction. Some leukotrienes can constrict the smooth muscles of the bronchial tube thirty times more effectively than histamine. In his book *The Zone,* Dr. Barry Sears points out that these mediators are actually hormones, *autocrine* hormones, and can also have an effect upon metabolism.

This is "classical" allergy, and its etiology is well un-derstood. Doctors are quite happy when they have a ra-tional scientific explanation for why something happens. This pathway (IgE) is the major but not the only way in which mast cells and basophils can be triggered; other nonspecific factors can also cause histamine release. As such, laboratory tests that are able to quantify the amount of allergen-specific IgE antibodies in the blood are fairly reliable (but not perfect) at identifying relevant allergens. Skin testing is also still in use. Some experts feel that it is more reliable; it may be, but it is certainly less convenient. Once the allergens have been identified, allergists commonly want to administer "shots" in the hope of achieving *desensitization.*

The History of Vaccination

Shots, also known as allergy vaccines, have an interesting history. The idea behind a vaccination is this: That which doesn't kill you makes you stronger. A fundamental prac-tice in modern medicine and public health, vaccination against specific infectious diseases has its basis in the observations of ancient thinkers, but was resisted by the scientific community when put into practice much later. Thucydides, an ancient Greek historian and chronicler of the Peloponnesian Wars, took note of the fact that victims of the plague in Athens did not succumb to the infection a second time if they survived their initial bout.

He wrote: "Yet still the ones who felt most pity were those who had had the plague themselves and had recovered from it. They knew what it was like and at the same time felt themselves to be safe, for no one caught the disease twice, or, if he did the second attack was never fatal." To a modern-day physician this observation makes perfect sense. We now accept that the immune system will mount a defense against a pathogen, such as a virus or a bacterium, by producing antibodies against it. The immune response might take a week to kick in, and during that time the victim may perish. However, if he or she survives, the immune system will immediately "recognize" the pathogen on subsequent exposures and will mount an attack much more quickly and effectively.

Although the credit for the "discovery" of vaccination against an infectious disease, in this case smallpox, is usually given to Dr. Edward Jenner, a cruder method was extant in India, Persia, and China as far back as the sixteenth century. Based on the observation that this often-fatal disease—which by the seventeenth century in England had replaced bubonic plague as the most fearsome and ravaging of all epidemics—rarely struck twice, the Orientals, in a process known as "ingrafting," would introduce a small quantity of the infected material (taken from pustules of a person stricken with the disease) into the person seeking to avoid it. By so inducing a mild form of the smallpox, the stimulation of the immune response would usually prevent a full-blown case from erupting. The method of introduction was either through the nose or by scratching the surface of the skin and applying it there.

The wife of the British ambassador to Constantinople in the early part of the eighteenth century, Lady Mary Montague, was so convinced of the benefits of ingrafting that she had her own children undergo the process. She wrote back to England regarding the effectiveness of the immunizing vaccine but also expressed concern that it would not be taken up by the English medical establishment. "I should not fail to write to some of our doctors very particularly about it, if I knew any of them that I thought had virtue enough to destroy such a considerable branch of their revenue for the good of mankind . . . Perhaps if I return, I may, however, have courage to war with them."

Jenner later observed that the milk maidens exposed to cowpox (a mild form of the disease), as evidenced by cowpox scars on their hands, did not succumb to smallpox, and did not develop smallpox scars on their face. It is now known that similar viruses cause both diseases and that unintentional inoculation against the one, through natural exposure, could—and did—provide immunity against the other.

In keeping with the tradition of organized medicine to resist any new way of thinking, the Royal Society rejected Jenner's work, declining to publish his findings for many years until 1798, when more studies were undertaken. No one knows how many people died unnecessarily in the meantime. However, this discovery marked a major paradigm shift and turning point in medical thought. Evidence for this shift is that the first Nobel Prize in medicine was awarded to Dr. Emil von Behring in 1901 for his work in developing an antitoxin effective against the childhood disease diphtheria. Some further attempts to develop immunization for specific diseases did not pan out, while others, particularly the efforts of

Louis Pasteur during the latter part of the nineteenth century, did.

No doubt, all these developments in vaccinations around the turn of the century gave rise to allergists experimenting with the same principles in an attempt to treat allergy. Based on the notion that inoculations with small but increasing doses of the offending allergen will eventually induce tolerance to the allergen, allergists began giving allergy shots. Never mind that the underlying cause of allergy is entirely different from the cause of infectious disease. Allergists at the time, lacking a scientific basis for and understanding of a mechanism of action, began this practice about one hundred years ago and continue it today. An allergy is not the result of an infectious agent, nor caused by a toxin derived from the agent that overwhelms the immune system. It is the result of the immune system overreacting to something that is not inherently harmful. The symptoms are brought on by the reaction of the immune system itself! Where is the logic?

Actually, recent understandings about how the immune system develops tolerance to the body's own proteins while the T lymphocytes are maturing has shed light on the possible development of effective allergy vaccines in the near future. However, the "shots" that a conventional allergist administers represent a rather crude approach that is rarely effective. A recent study reported in the prestigious *New England Journal of Medicine* shows that shots are of no significant benefit as compared with a placebo when it comes to treating children with asthma. Why are allergy shots still used? Contrast this with the treatment indicated for a diagnosis of food sensitivity— mere avoidance of the offending foods. One can readily see the economic advantage for the allergist to continue to give and charge for weekly shots rather than give dietary advice once. The answer may lie more within economics than within science.

Intolerance, the Other Allergic Reaction

Besides the classical food allergy reaction within our body, we need to look at another problem that can develop within the body's suit of armor. Though less instantaneous, and often less obvious, this reaction is no less destructive and *is* much more common. This occurs when the cells attack one or more common foods either through a similar chemical assault or through some other defensive strategy. Rather than impacting the system instantaneously, the defense mechanisms take a slower but no less deliberate route. The effects produce delayed reactions in the body, perhaps several hours or even days later—thereby rendering diagnosis by patient history or conventional allergy testing extremely difficult or impossible. This process begins when a person eats a food or ingests a chemical or drug that does not agree with the body. This kink in the body's defense systems is known as an intolerance.

As mentioned earlier, a small number of us have "true" food allergies in which the body reacts in a predictable fashion—with an immune system attack that results in symptoms such as sneezing, coughing, or a skin rash. For the multitudes who have food intolerance, explanations for their symptoms, such as fatigue, migraines, arthritis, and obesity, are not so straightforward. The disruption in the system could arise from an inappropriate immune system response (although a slightly different one than in the case of "true" food allergy). The result, arising from digestive, enzymatic, or hormonal disruptions, is overload of one or more detoxification pathways. It may involve the pharmacological-mediated effects of chemicals naturally occurring in or added to the food.

Indeed, food intolerance may well be the most misunderstood health issue today. Conventional doctors often do not accept it, and occasionally hold a professional bias against it.

Food Intolerance: Hard to Swallow?

Because food intolerance wasn't taught in medical school, many doctors consider it irrelevant. This raises an interesting point: Large pharmaceutical companies exert a subtle but significant influence on medical school curricula. In fact, drug companies continue to influence a physician throughout his or her career. Consider this comment from the Public Citizen Health Research Group in Britain regarding drug company influence on medical education:

> Thus, a student may first listen to a patient's heart with a stethoscope provided by Eli Lilly & Co. He or she may learn to recognize the different heart sounds by listening to tape recordings from the school library, featuring the various sounds made by a healthy heart, interspersed with the words "Merck Sharp and Dohme" at frequent intervals. He or she may study with the aid of a series of well-illustrated handbooks on various medical subjects, a gift from the Upjohn Co., or look up strange new words in a medical dictionary from Sandoz, Inc. When the young doctor is in the last years of medical school and begins practical training, he or she may enjoy anything from pocket notebooks from CIBA Pharmaceutical Company to doughnuts and pizza parties provided by other drug companies. All of this helps to create a favorable image of the drug company on the mind of the young doctor.

Dr. Charles Atkins confirms this relationship between doctors and drug companies in the February 9,

1998, issue of *American Medical News:* "For years, [doctors] and the drug companies have been reinforcing the hell out of each other; and if it wasn't for legal restrictions, they'd give [doctors] things much better than expensive pens." To generalize, drug companies by and large don't like the work done in the area of food intolerance; that is because food intolerance could have a big impact on their profits. The following story best illustrates this point: Kahlil Gibran, the Persian poet, best known for his poem *The Prophet,* wrote a short story about a priest traveling in the forest, who one day happened upon none other than Lucifer himself. As fate would have it, Lucifer had somehow suffered a terrible accident and his injuries would surely cause his death if he were not to receive timely medical assistance. Ironically, the priest was his only hope for survival—if only he could convince the priest to carry him to the town. Of course, no self-respecting God-fearing priest would do such a thing; in fact, Lucifer's grim circumstances would be cause for great jubilation.

Nonetheless, Lucifer's power of persuasion is not to be underestimated, even regarding those whose sworn duty is for the good of mankind—or so the story goes. At first the priest demurred, wanting nothing to do with any type of rescue. Then Lucifer pointed out to the priest that if he were to die, the entire source of all that was evil and tempting to mankind that kept men and women from practicing their religion, would die along with him. And while that at first might seem the very fulfillment of religion and a great thing overall, it would also mean that things would change. "Without the fear of the devil and a lifetime in hell, would the people still need the Church and the Priesthood?" said Lucifer. Perhaps not; and if not, the priest would be out of a job. He would no longer be able to live off the alms from the people and would have to seek a new form of employment—not an attractive proposition. The priest rationalized that the potential downfall of the church (and therefore his privileged position in society) was too much to risk. The priest then carried Lucifer into town, where the devil's wounds got the needed attention, leaving him alive and well. No one was the wiser and the priest kept his job.

Intolerant of Food Intolerance

A senior representative from a major American health-care provider was offered an opportunity to include the ALCAT Test in their services. She declined the opportunity, a move that would have prevented a lot of illness and saved the health-care system substantial sums of money. Much like the priest in the story above, the representative stated that "our hospitals make a lot of money treating sick people."

Value of Test Confirmed

However, researchers in South Africa recently completed an outcome study. It confirms the cost-effectiveness of using the ALCAT Test for food and chemical sensitivities to pinpoint the cause of many common medical problems, including migraine, allergy, irritability, arthritis, chronic fatigue, chronic sinusitis, spastic colon, irritable bowel syndrome, obesity, eczema, and acne. Patients were tested, then counseled regarding dietary elimination of test-positive foods and additives. Three to six months later an independent research organization interviewed a random selection of patients to assess the degree of improvement in self-reported disease symptoms. A scale of zero to five was used with zero representing no improvement, three showing improvement, and five representing total cure. Of the subjects, 274 had multiple symptoms. Most symptom categories showed dramatic improvement. The following percentages reflect the number of respondents reporting a three, four, or five outcome in their respective conditions.

Acne	46%
Arthritis	77%
Chronic fatigue	71%
Chronic sinusitis	62%
Diarrhea/constipation	73%
Eczema	67%
Migraine	78%
Spastic colon	71%

These findings underscore the significance of cost savings for a wide range of disorders.

Dr. Geldenhuys, clinical consultant to the laboratory, where the ALCAT Test is performed, stated: "We've seen the dramatic improvement possible when sensitivities are accurately determined and the appropriate modification to diet is instituted. Using the ALCAT Test unquestionably resulted in health and monetary benefits for the majority of our patients."

Other studies support the view that an early diagnosis of food sensitivities can save the health-care system money. In 1990 Dr. Alison Bunnin of Oxford University reviewed a number of cost-benefit studies and found a significant benefit in terms of cost savings for drugs, hospitalizations, doctor's visits, and time lost from work and school. The same year, Dr. Jonathan Brostoff, immunologist at the Middlesex Hospital Medical School in London and consultant to the NHS, found that using the ALCAT Test in a cohort of 22 irritable bowel syndrome (IBS) patients represented a 92 percent cost savings when compared to the conventional form of drug treatment.

The economic impact of health problems associated with food or food additive sensitivity is escalating. The incidence of migraine has increased by nearly 60 percent in the U.S. in the last decade. Estimates of industry losses attributable to migraine sufferers' absenteeism and reduced productivity range from $6.5 billion to $17.2 billion annually. Irritable bowel syndrome affects nearly 20 percent of the U.S. population.

Notwithstanding the views of the ancient philosophers and physicians, such as Hippocrates, Lucretius, and others, who recognized that "one man's meat is another man's poison," the notion that otherwise healthy food can be the cause of disease is, in some respects, a new idea. For the reasons mentioned, it is not unusual for new ideas in medicine to be met with skepticism—and sometimes fervent and often irrational resistance. Such is the case with most major discoveries in the field of immunology and infectious diseases. Nowadays, every grammar school child knows that vitamin C, apart from its numerous other benefits, prevents scurvy. The idea first occurred to Dr. James Lind, who was physician to the British Navy in the middle of the eighteenth century. He conducted a controlled trial wherein sailors in one group were provided supplemental citrus fruit to their usual diet, while sailors in another group ate their standard fare. The results demonstrated that eating the citrus fruit conferred protection from scurvy, and Dr. Lind published his findings in 1753. However, it wasn't until 42 years later, in 1795, that his findings were accepted and limes were then routinely taken aboard Navy voyages, thus giving rise to the name "Limeys."

It is no surprise then that "classical" food allergy (that is, IgE–mediated, immediate symptom onset reactions) has usurped prominence over food intolerance, also known as "hidden" food allergy. Many biological mechanisms, both known and suspected, are involved in food intolerance. This further explains why no two people with food intolerance have exactly the same symptoms. Indeed, food intolerance is a complex subject involving a number of bodily processes and virtually any organ or combination of organs. Few generalizations can be made; however, certain features do characterize this type of food sensitivity, and distinguish it from classic food allergy.

As discussed in chapter 1, food intolerance is a delayed reaction to foods, unlike traditional food allergy, which causes immediate reaction from the body. The difference boils down to proof. When you eat peanuts and immediately get hives, the cause-and-effect relationship between your body and the food cannot be disputed. But when your symptoms cannot be directly tied to a food because they appear hours or days after you eat it, any skeptic can easily argue that the food is not causing the problems.

Classic allergy is understood to occur as the result of a breakdown in one mechanism of the body—the immune system; in food intolerance, the immune system may or may not be involved. Food intolerance can also be instigated by the absorption of toxic elements into the system or by the pharmacological (drug-like) reactions of certain chemicals in foods. What's more, intolerance can be perpetrated by a combination of mechanisms, and because one system in our body depends on another, the rest can topple like dominos when one is unhealthy. For example, overusing antibiotics can cause the lining of your intestines to become weak, thereby setting the stage for adverse immune reactions. However, whichever mechanisms are involved— the immune system, toxic overload, or pharmacological effects—the result is the same. The white blood cells, swollen and fragile from the influence of the particular allergenic food, react by releasing granules of chemicals to fight the invader. This effect, a final common pathway, can be easily measured with a simple blood test, the ALCAT Test.

Digestion: The Front Line to Good Health

Think of your body as a finely tuned engine with food as its fuel. To ensure that your body receives adequate fuel, your digestive system must first properly digest all food, including proteins, the most difficult molecules to digest—and it must deal with the unwanted non-nutrients and toxins that accompany all forms of food. The non-nutrient material and toxins, both naturally occurring and man-made, are dealt with in three ways:

- As the gut absorbs digested food, it will eliminate some chemicals.
- Some toxins will be absorbed and travel to the liver, a major detoxifying organ.
- Other non-nutrient matter will be absorbed into the white cell population of the immune system for elimination.

The nutrients in foods are not ready-to-use. They first must be broken down by digestion into a suitable size for absorption into the system. Then they must be properly absorbed into the bloodstream so they can be transported to the cells, where they are needed for energy, building, and repair. It is largely believed that undigested proteins, carbohydrates, and fats (and even yeast cells) can be absorbed into the bloodstream, where they can cause allergic reactions. Good digestion requires a carefully coordinated series of mechanical and biochemical reactions.

When everything is running correctly, proper digestion begins in the mouth with thorough chewing. Grinding the food with the teeth begins the mechanical breakdown of a meal. Saliva triggers the start of the chemical breakdown. It contains enzymes that start the digestion of carbohydrates. In the stomach, adequate amounts of hydrochloric acid and pepsin (a protein-digesting enzyme) are needed to break down dietary proteins. Once food moves to the small intestine, hydrochloric acid and other factors trigger the pancreas to release special enzymes. These acids and enzymes break down food into basic nutrients—vitamins, minerals, carbohydrates, fats, water, protein (amino acids), and essential trace elements—which are absorbed by billions of *villi* (tiny projections) in the small intestine.

If foods, especially proteins, have not been properly digested due to insufficient hydrochloric acid (often a result of food intolerance), not only is the food incompletely digested and improperly sterilized, but this condition sets up a chain reaction. When food reaches the pancreas in a low-acid state, the pancreas produces fewer of the bicarbonates and digestive enzymes necessary to alkalize the food. When the food components are not digested, your immune system does not recognize them as nutritional and beneficial, and it responds protectively by producing antibodies. This starts a series of defensive reactions, which can affect many tissues and organs, including the cardiovascular system. The result can be a multitude of symptoms depending on the tissue or organ affected.

Nutrients in food are absorbed into the bloodstream by both the small and large intestines. Food that isn't digested completely will not be absorbed through a healthy intestinal lining. But, if stress, chemicals, or disease compromises the intestinal mucosa, incompletely digested food macromolecules may be absorbed into the bloodstream. Finally, in the intestinal tract, billions of friendly bacteria aid with digestion, vitamin production, and immune defense. In some people, the delicate balance of friendly to non-friendly bacteria can be disrupted due to many factors, including a prolonged use of antibiotics, steroids, or hormone pills, an overgrowth of *candida albicans* or parasites, or a diet high in fat and sugar.

As we can see from this brief snapshot of the intricate and continuous digestive process, at any point along the complex route something can go wrong. A malfunction means, for one thing, that we're not properly absorbing all the nutrients we're eating, which, if this continues over time, results in malnutrition. Also, the lack of proper nutrition, along with a continual bombardment of incompletely digested foods into the bloodstream, will impact proper functioning of the powerful and complex immune system, which is our body's barrier to the foreign substances in the world. If this occurs, it leaves the body vulnerable to many health problems, including food intolerance.

Enzymes: The Labor Force of the Body

Enzymes are specialized types of protein molecules that are essential to life. Although they are so small they can't even be seen under a microscope, thousands of different enzymes inhabit the human body. Because enzymes are needed for every chemical action and reaction in the body, they do a tremendous amount of work. For example, digestive enzymes digest all of our food, creating particles small enough to pass through the intestines into the bloodstream. They break down food so that its energy can be used to build muscles, nerves, blood, and hormones; assist in storing sugar in the liver and muscles; and turn fat into fatty tissue. Detoxification enzymes break down toxins in the blood and tissues, rendering them harmless. Many experts in allergy and food intolerance believe that defective or deficient enzymes play a part in food intolerance.

The human body is not maintained by mere food intake, but rather by what it successfully digests. As discussed, the more digestion that takes place before the food reaches the small intestine, the better for the integrity, strength, and immunity of the whole body. Basically, the symptoms of allergy are the body's attempt to resist the organisms, toxins, and foods that are likely to damage tissues and organs. The white blood cells of the immune system help destroy allergenic substances and other toxins by engulfing them and digesting or partially destroying their substances, making it easier for the body to eliminate them. In most cases, they do this by secreting detoxification enzymes, which help break down the allergenic substances. These enzymatic activities fail in some people for a variety of reasons. Without the quick and effective action of these enzymes, toxins increase and spread quickly throughout the body, causing or continuing the development of food intolerance and its many accompanying physical problems and symptoms.

An individual's enzyme makeup is largely hereditary, with all the necessary information encoded in the genes. The lack of a particular enzyme or the presence of a defective enzyme is often handed down from parent to child. Intolerance to a particular food or foods could be related to the fact that one's ancestors were never exposed to that food, so never developed a genetic predisposition to deal with it enzymatically. For example, vast numbers of indigenous populations lack the enzyme to digest cow's milk because their ancestors were never exposed to cow's milk and, genetically speaking, had no need to develop the necessary enzymes to digest milk. Also, a person can develop a deficiency of a particular enzyme due to several factors, including inadequate nutrition, stress, chemical bombardment, and illness.

The Immune System: The Body's Bodyguard

A great, dramatic war is taking place in our bodies around the clock. Without this continuous war we would die, because our bodies have many powerful enemies—billions of bacteria, viruses, parasites, and other microorganisms and toxins that invade our system at any given moment. But our body has an even more powerful system for dealing with these potential troublemakers—our immune system. A strong immune system is essential to protect us from disease and to promote well-being. It could take volumes to fully describe our complex and dynamic immune system. We'll instead give you a summary of how the system works, and where our suit of armor can break down with regard to allergy and food intolerance, thereby producing rather than protecting our bodies against disease.

An extensive cast of characters is involved in the intricate drama that protects the body from foreigners. A diverse army of specialized blood cells and molecules work in concert, continually communicating with each other to further create, defend, and destroy. Several types of white blood cells (leukocytes), such as lymphocytes, macrophages, T cells, B cells, and neutrophils comprise a major part of the immune-system players. (As mentioned before, T cells get their name from the thymus gland that aids in their production; B cells are named for bone marrow, where they are formed.) Although T cells and B cells are both lymphocytes, they differ slightly in their duties. T lymphocytes become sensitized to specific toxins or antigens (substances that cause immune responses) and attack them whenever they enter the body. B lymphocytes produce antibodies, the molecules that react with and aid in the destruction of certain allergenic substances in the body.

The ultimate targets of all immune responses are "antigens," usually foreign molecules from bacteria, viruses, parasites, or other toxic invaders. The immune system's goal is to clear the antigens from the body. Specialized immune cells, such as macrophages, serve as the first line of defense, roaming the body, ingesting the antigens, and fragmenting them into tiny pieces. These pieces are joined to special molecules and displayed on their surface, like prisoners placed in stocks in the Town Square for all to see. A complex series of chemical communications takes place with the goal of informing specialized B cells about the identity of the prisoners already captured so that they can identify and immobilize any similar criminals not yet captured. After receiving the message, the B cells divide into plasma cells, which secrete "antibody" proteins. These antibodies (a protein molecule that helps combat disease-causing bacteria, viruses, and allergens) go about the task of binding to all antigens they find, like cops handcuffing themselves to prisoners. The antibodies can then neutralize the antigens or help facilitate their destruction by enlisting the aid of complement proteins (defense proteins in the blood) or scavenger (eating) cells called phagocytes. The five main types of fighting antibodies, also known as isotypes or immunoglobulin (Ig for short) are IgE, IgG, IgA, IgM, and IgD.

The primary antibody involved in classic allergy (also known as "immediate hypersensitivity") is IgE, which acts somewhat differently than the rest. When allergic individuals with classic food allergy eat certain foods, their immune system is alerted to make IgE antibodies specific to that food. Then millions of these highly specialized IgE antibodies circulate in the blood, binding to the surface of basophils (cells that float in the blood) and entering the body tissues, where they attach themselves to the surface of mast cells. Mast cells are found imbedded in the body's solid tissues at sites where the body comes into contact with the environment such as the lungs, the nasal passages, and the intestinal walls. Basophils and mast cells produce and store the chemical mediators that do so much damage to allergenic individuals.

This chemical arsenal, stored in tiny membrane-bound packets, includes histamines, inflammatory prostaglandins, leukotrienes, heparin, serotonin, and others. When these chemicals get the signal, they burst out of the cells and begin causing major changes in the cells and tissues to which they have attached. Each potent chemical (called a mediator, because it mediates change) has its own particular effect on the body—much like a soldier who specializes in air, ground, or water missions. Some make blood vessels open up, others make them leakier so that blood escapes through the vessel wall, and several chemicals make the smooth muscles of our lungs, stomach, intestines, and bladder contract. In other words, they cause sneezing, coughing, diarrhea, and other such symptoms. The packets of chemicals give the cells a granular appearance, so the process in which they react and release the chemicals is called degranulation. The action doesn't stop there. Among the results of the chain reaction started by the mast cell degranulation is inflammation, which causes phagocytes (all-purpose defense cells),

---

The food intolerant person is not given the warning that enables the victim of classic food allergy to avoid the problem-causing food.

---

including macrophages ("big eaters"), to engulf and destroy unwanted invaders.

This system is powerful and keeps us healthy in a world of otherwise completely destructive invaders. However, there is one bug in the system—in individuals who develop food intolerance, something goes wrong and causes cracks to develop in the body's defense mechanism. While degranulation of the chemical mediators is instantaneous in food allergy, food intolerance rarely causes an instant reaction. Rather, the immune system begins a slow but steady dance of destruction involving one or more systems of the body and producing one or more health problems. The food intolerant person is not given the warning that enables the victim of classic food allergy to avoid the problem-causing food. So the bombardment of the immune system and other malfunctions continues relentlessly. To further complicate diagnosis, an immune process known as neurogenic switching explains how a stimulus at one site of the body can lead to inflammation at another site. The result is frequently chronic, vague, low-grade symptoms.

Furthermore, food can trigger an immune reaction in several ways, which contributes to the difficulty of diagnosing food intolerance. Some foods are believed to contain substances that trigger mast cells directly, as do toxins produced by some bacteria. It's also thought that the body may trigger mast cell degranulation directly in response to an irritant substance in food. Hypersensitivity to a food develops when the same antigen repeatedly assaults the immune system. The system, like a computer, has a powerful memory. When an organism is encountered for the second or third time, the defenses are marshaled quickly so that the organism does not have the chance to multiply and cause disease. In other words, our body strategizes a specific immune defense against a possible future invasion by the same antigen. Once this has happened, the person will likely be sensitive to this food for the rest of his or her life.

How can all of this damage occur without our knowing? The majority of food allergy reactions are silent, insidious, and chronic for one simple reason: They take place in the tissues and organs that do not perceive pain or discomfort. Thus, chronic immune assaults can go on daily with no recognized symptoms until our body finally is overwhelmed and develops chronic symptoms.

One final note on the relationship of food intolerance and the immune system: Not only does overreaction of the immune system to particular foods wreak havoc on a food intolerant person's health, but depletion of the immune system due to chronic overreaction taxes the body's natural defense system. This leaves us vulnerable to the effects of other harmful invaders. A weakened, overworked immune system alone is enough to make us very sick.

Metabolic Stress and Overload

Many symptoms of food intolerance are due to an overloaded metabolic system. In other words, for one or more of various reasons, the amount of offending foods, including their nutrients and accompanying non-nutrients, have exceeded the body's ability to metabolize them. In particular, if the non-nutrients, which are ingested along with the nutrients, are allowed to accumulate, they quickly become toxic and result in many diverse symptoms. Normally, these symptoms are temporary; the body recovers when the offending foods and chemicals are withdrawn for awhile.

Impacting this metabolism of offending foods and toxins is each person's unique inherited "metabolic rate." About 25 percent of the population has a faster metabolism than normal and another 25 percent has a slower rate—as much as 11 times slower, which can lead to serious trouble, as you'll see. The source of the metabolic rate is one of the body's critical pathways within the cells, called the "cytochrome P450 system," upon which about eight or nine of the pathways of detoxification and elimination must depend.

When this powerful and unique system is faulty, it limits the metabolic rates of many other cellular pathways. Other systems that extract nutrients from food can accelerate according to the nutrient concentration, and thereby efficiently extract what the body needs for building and repair, but the cytochrome P450 system cannot accelerate. It has a fixed rate of metabolism and therefore cannot speed up to deal with an overload. Instead, it must choose what non-nutrient substrates in the system it will eliminate, since it cannot eliminate them all.

For example, in a slow metabolizer, a cup of coffee at dinner may keep them awake into the wee hours of the morning, whereas those with normal cytochrome P450 systems will have cleared the caffeine by midnight and be soundly asleep. Another example of the concept of "rate of metabolism" is alcohol. When most of us consume alcohol at the rate of one average drink per hour, we can go for days without intoxication, because the body is able to metabolize it at this rate. The body has a fixed rate of metabolism for alcohol and other substances, a so-called "zero order" rate, above which is impossible to accelerate; consequently ingestion must be limited to levels that can be metabolized.

To back up this drawback in metabolic rate, the body may call into service the white blood cells of the immune system to help clean up the spillover. As mentioned earlier, special white blood cells will bind to the offending substances and hold them in a neutral state until the liver can detoxify them. Unfortunately, our bodies have no shortage of non-nutrients with which we must contend. The myriad of non-nutrients that we need to detoxify is increased ever more by modern agriculture, food preservation, and cooking methods. So the probability of overload exists for everyone, whether their cytochrome P450 system metabolizes quickly, normally, or slowly.

When chronic food intolerance exists in the body, the immune system's defense system is in constant attack mode, firing its chemical weapons on a regular basis to neutralize the enemy.

Another aspect to overload is that when too many variables impact our lives—poor diet, stress, and environmental pollution, for example—we overload our systems. Something has to give. Sometimes we can deal with the overload, but pile on too many troubles and we can quickly overtax our system.

The Structure and Function of the Gut

Under normal, healthy conditions, the one-eighth-inch-thick mucosal membrane barrier that lines the intestinal wall allows only completely digested protein to pass into the bloodstream. This membrane is all that stands between the intestinal tract—the body's elimination system—and the bloodstream. When this barrier is breached, it develops gaps or leaks that get bigger and make the lining more permeable. This leaves us wide open for assorted health problems. This condition, known as "leaky gut," permits the partially digested large food macromolecules (and perhaps microorganisms, enterotoxins, and drugs) to enter the bloodstream and disturb its efficient functioning. Incompletely digested proteins are not nutrients. As mentioned earlier, those that reach the bloodstream are viewed as aliens and the body sends out an army of antibodies to take care of the enemies. The system's overreaction can lead to localized inflammation in the gut. Some evidence suggests that people with food intolerance have leakier gut walls than people without food intolerance, so more undigested food molecules get through.

If incompletely digested foods do reach the bloodstream, antibodies quickly attach themselves to the oversized macromolecules, effectively tagging them for cleanup by specialized white blood cells. However, when the white blood cells have too many complexes to clean up, the food molecules may overwhelm the cleanup crew. These clusters of antibodies and proteins, called circulating immune complexes (CICs), travel through the bloodstream until they are eventually dumped just about anywhere in the body, including the joints, muscles, skin, organs, and lungs. This dumping attracts immune cells and other proteins, leading to inflammation, pain, wheezing, fatigue, water retention, weight gain, poor immunity, coughing, sneezing, and other symptoms.

The integrity of the gut wall is made more permeable by a variety of conditions, including poor nutrition, overuse of antibiotics or other medications, alcohol, a viral infection, a *candida* overgrowth, and health problems. What's more, the immune system's overreaction to allergens—specifically the potent chemical mediators discharged by the mast cells—is also thought to create damaging long-range consequences on this mucosal lining. When chronic food intolerance exists in the body, the immune system's defense system is in constant attack mode, firing its chemical weapons on a regular basis to neutralize the enemy. This constant release of powerful (and often painful) chemical mediators from the mast cells upsets the delicate balance in the digestive system. This unhealthy situation continues a self-perpetuating cycle that becomes a cascade of chronic disease.

Individual Biochemistry:
No "One Size Fits All" Diet

Just as no single mechanism lies behind all food intolerance, no two people with food intolerance are the same. For one thing, an aspect of genetics, called genetic polymorphism, affects all types of reactions that might be associated with symptoms caused by food. Genetic polymorphism is what makes each of us different, despite the fact that our genetic makeup is almost identical. This means that distinct types of factors are uniquely common to a group of people within the human race—for example, Mediterraneans, or Eskimos. These groups have different enzymes or enzymes that operate at a unique rate. If your ancestors were never exposed to a particular food, it's likely you and others in your group never developed a genetic predisposition to deal with it enzymatically. As such, it has been discovered that different groups will react to food, its metabolism, and its toxicity in different ways.

What's more, within these groups, each individual's biochemistry is completely unique. Although primarily inherited, it is also affected by environment, lifestyle, health, and other experiences. As such, each person with food intolerance has different symptoms, which vary in degree, age of onset, duration, location, and amount of food needed to trigger the symptoms. The same food can produce vastly different symptoms in different people, and different foods can cause different symptoms in the same person. So, before you have eaten even one mouthful of food, several scenarios are possible. These factors explain why no one single diet will fit every person's nutritional and health needs. Only an individualized diet, which eliminates your intolerant foods, will help ensure that allergens and toxins that interfere with maximum health do not overload your system.

When we are sick, something in the body is wrong. It's clear from this brief explanation the multitude of problems that can occur in our digestive system, immune system, and enzymatic system. Preventative medical doctors agree that when any one of these systems are not working a person has taken a step further away from optimal health. The aim of maximum health is to get these processes and others working at optimum performance. Once you get these systems healthy, you've taken a giant step to enabling your body to use these dynamic and powerful systems to take care of itself. Clearly, if you remove food to which you are intolerant, you'll give your body a fighting chance to clear up the migraines, joint pains, excess weight, and other health problems triggered and compounded by foods. Identifying and removing reactive foods is the key to your good health.

CHAPTER 5

Overweight: As American As Apple Pie

Contemporary medicine seeks to satisfy the needs and demands of an ever-growing population of overweight Americans by prescribing drugs that work on appetite suppression, serotonin levels, and the binding of fat in the intestine. Although many studies suggest these treatments work, we still treat obesity blindly. Few patients are getting well, and we don't know why people are getting more and more overweight.

The following statement from the *Journal of the American Medical Association* (Vol. 272, No. 3, July 20, 1994) summarizes the results of four separate large national studies pertaining to obesity.

> Understanding the underlying reasons for the increased prevalence of overweight in the United States and elucidating the potential consequences for health outcomes challenge our understanding of the etiology, treatment, and prevention of overweight. Overweight is increasing in U.S. adults and continues to be a public health dilemma for

which no efficacious, practical, and long-lasting preventive
or therapeutic solution has yet been identified.

Why Overweight?

At the disposal of every American is the "food pyramid,"
put forth by the agriculture department as the appropriate proportions of fats, proteins, and carbohydrates to
keep us healthy. Healthy perhaps, but it certainly won't
trim our waistline. Endless studies show that eating too
much will cause weight gain, more studies show that taking medication causes weight loss, and even more en-
lightening studies prove if one changes what he does he
won't do it any more (lifestyle change). Give me a break!
Of all the diseases, obesity would seem obviously due to
an abnormal reaction to food. The clue is that in spite of
all the theories, Americans continue to gain weight.

Whether alone or in conjunction, accepted therapies for overweight often don't work for the long term.
Their weakness lies in the inaccurate premise that every
individual is identical in digestion, metabolism, and function. If this were true, why aren't we all presidents? The
fact is that in spite of all the scientific study and analysis,
humans defy general categorization. Each of us differs in
the way we respond to food, oxygen, chemicals, and even
visual and sensory input. We are as different in our reaction to foods as in our political philosophies.

The documented biochemical progression of food
through our bodies does not explain our overweight or
abnormal cravings for food. We don't have the full picture; we're overlooking some factor. To date the great
majority of research has been directed toward developing
medications to treat symptoms of hunger and cravings.
Given the incredible amount of money to be made in the

field of antiobesity medication—to help people lose the same pound of fat over and over—why would drug companies spend money researching the role of food intolerance? Which among them is going to shoot the goose laying the golden eggs?

Dr. Donna Ryan, M.D., states that "more than one in three Americans are overweight . . . up from one in four Americans a little more than a decade earlier." We must agree with her conclusion:

> One would think that the emphasis on managed care would spur a reassessment of the need for preventative approaches. Obesity contributes directly and indirectly to chronic disease risk, and measures to ameliorate and prevent the disorder should receive top priority for research funding.
>
> —"Medicating the Obese Patient," *Endocrinology and Metabolism Clinics of North America*, vol. 25, no. 4, Dec. 1996

The relationship of food intolerance to overweight is like the relationship of gasoline to fire: Gasoline may cause the fire and will surely keep it raging. So suggestive is the relationship that I routinely recommend that persons with a history of "yo-yo dieting" get tested for food intolerance. Furthermore, if overweight patients have concurrent symptoms associated with food sensitivities, testing is even more imperative. If food intolerance is what has kept them sick or caused the regain of weight, they need to know this before they can hope to keep off the weight. And avoiding foods is much safer than taking medication for the long term.

The Serotonin Made Me Do It

Finally a logical explanation for the heretofore uncontrollable desire to eat inappropriate foods at inappropriate times has surfaced: You crave chocolate tonight because of your allergic response to the carrots you ate yesterday. Simply put, the allergic reaction resulted in a depletion of serotonin in your system. Responding to your brain's flashing red warning lights of low serotonin, you subconsciously search out foods to increase brain serotonin levels.

"Wait a minute!" the enlightened among you may cry, "How can eating chocolate, a carbohydrate, cause an increase in a protein hormone in the brain?" At the risk of losing the thought at hand, this may be the time to clarify how serotonin fits into this picture. Serotonin is produced on-site in the brain. It cannot get into the brain from the bloodstream. To produce serotonin, the brain must have precursors in the form of certain amino acid–building blocks. Amino acids are the smallest building blocks that the body uses to make proteins it needs as hormones. The specific precursor to serotonin is tryptophan.

Tryptophan is special in that it is pretty scarce in the bloodstream. Most other amino acids are branched chain amino acids and are fairly plentiful compared to tryptophan. At any rate, all these amino acids line up at the blood-brain barrier waiting their turn to be transported to the brain. The blood-brain barrier is like the border between countries. The body is very particular as to what gets through the blood-brain barrier, and a backup develops. Meanwhile the level of serotonin in the brain continues to fall. Your brain tells you to go eat something sweet. As soon as you do that, your insulin level soars.

The immediate effect of insulin in the bloodstream is to direct all the branched chain amino acids to their respective posts to begin building muscle and enzymes to take advantage of the sugary energy you have just eaten. The insulin sweeps through all the amino acids in line at the blood-brain barrier, conscripting all those that are branched chain amino acids for duties elsewhere in the body. Tryptophan, normally not one of the more common amino acids, now finds itself highly concentrated at the blood-brain barrier by virtue of the insulin tidal wave.

Subsequently more tryptophan enters the brain more quickly and is promptly converted to serotonin, one of the neurotransmitters responsible for determining hunger. As serotonin levels rise, the need to feed disappears and the body assumes a well-fed, calm, peaceful state. As serotonin levels decay, this process repeats itself. The whole process is thrown into action each and every time serotonin levels drop below a certain set point for that individual. External factors may also cause a depletion of serotonin. These include long-term stress, sleep deprivation, illness, and food-sensitivity reactions. Regardless of the precipitating event, the bodily urge to raise serotonin levels manifests as a strong craving for a food that will raise insulin levels and replenish serotonin levels rapidly. This is why you crave sweets.

Down Insulin! Down! Bad Insulin!

One chemical reaction in the body leads to another in perpetual motion. Serotonin aside, we now have raging insulin levels as the body tries to take advantage of the precious sugar energy you have consumed. Insulin will direct the blood glucose (sugar) into the muscle cells and liver, where it can be stored for future use as glycogen. You are unlikely to need it immediately because of your current drowsy state resulting from elevated serotonin levels. Not one to waste energy resources, the body will direct the conversion of excess glucose into fat once all the storage capacity for glycogen is filled. Coincidentally, the effect of insulin is to open the fat cell to accept fat for storage and close off the release of fat from the cell into the bloodstream. This is because the body will preferentially use glucose as an energy source over fat, when it is available. This is a good example of what is called a cascade.

The end result is that you are lethargic with a full tank of energy stored as both glycogen and fat. Since your serotonin level is fine, your only tendency to eat is from a fluctuating insulin level causing you to seek sweets to correct your hypoglycemia.

This is a nightmare of perpetual bad news for the overweight patient. Elevated serotonin levels and intermittent hypoglycemia keep one lethargic while increased insulin levels promote storing more energy as fat. You can tell right now, the scales are not going to be kind tomorrow!

Yes, food sensitivities can keep you fat. If you are someone who exercises regularly, eats "right," and still can't lose weight, think about the possibility that you may have food sensitivities. You may try to avoid sugary sweets, but probably liberally indulge in pasta, bread, or starches. The body is responding to the lowered serotonin levels resulting from a delayed food sensitivity. These refined grain products may in some cases raise insulin levels as fast or faster than sugar. Compound the dilemma by eating any amount of saturated fat along with your sugar or refined grain treat and stand back. Those fat cells are going to swell. Finding out whether you have a food intolerance that leads you to crave carbohydrates can enable you to put an end to the vicious cycle. Eliminating your reactive foods will result in diminished cravings and a proper resumption of normal metabolic pathways. Weight loss will then follow this normalizing of body functions.

The Agony of "The Feed"

It may sound obvious, but still bears saying: "It's not fun being overweight." I don't know anyone who has said, "Yeah, I think I will totally ignore myself until I weigh 350 pounds." Since this is not one of those noble goals we set for ourselves in high school, it is by default a negative aspect of our adult development. The fact is that the pain and anguish start early as one gains weight. Initially, the pain is one of depriving oneself of food as a pleasure from time to time to control small weight gains. Panic and fear follow this, as short-term dieting no longer does the job. Short-term successes with "quick-fix" medication lead to long-term disgust as the pounds come back. Soon denial and guilt obstruct effective treatment. Self-esteem falls off the edge of the table and depression darkens life. Psychologically, some people may resign themselves to their condition, remaining fat and possibly desexualizing themselves. Those you know who are overweight have or will feel each of these emotions as they slowly withdraw from activities and events they enjoy. Despite their other successes, they live in the shadow of defeat until they get over this final hurdle. Understand their frustration. After all, they were never voted "most likely to be fat."

Doom and Gloom

As we try to lose weight, we unconsciously doom success as we approach each weight-loss effort with short-term goals. Perhaps the goals are left from the days when the pounds fell away easily or perhaps stem from denial that we have a serious problem with food. At any rate, we secretly realize that this weight problem is forever. We've read everywhere that more than 90 percent of those who lose weight gain it back within a year or two. We accept our fate and open our wallets. Desperate to at least give the appearance of making an effort to get the weight off, we proceed from one weight-loss gimmick to another. Some actually work for a short period, but the weight always finds its way back. In this way we shield ourselves from open criticism that we are weak, or that we just don't care about ourselves.

Fair-weather Friends

People close to us seem to flaunt our weakness as they offer food in abundance. Confused as to what would really make us happy, our friends offer the gift we obviously enjoy. Unwilling to bring attention to ourselves, we eat, begrudgingly fitting into the very mold society cast for us. Once started, we now eat to elevate ourselves from the pit of self-pity and guilt with a serotonin surge. We have a disease. No other illness is treated with such callous disregard by society.

If you are someone who exercises regularly, eats "right," and still can't lose weight, think about the possibility that you may have food sensitivities.

We are dying and no one cares. Others in fact take every opportunity to make money off our misfortune. They tempt us with stories of success and pass us off to the next "90-day wonder" program, knowing we will return. Even many of our doctors don't seem to realize we are sick. We have a ravaging chemical reaction coursing through our bodies and don't know why. Food sensitivities leading to absorptive malnutrition, immune system dysfunction, and multiple organ system symptoms brand us as "chronic disease patients." In the case of allergic reaction to foods, the effect on the body is similar to that of a parasite, which drains the host's reserves of energy, creates imbalances in brain chemistry, and interrupts desirable body functions. To try to keep up nutritionally with this constant drain and waste of body energy would be like trying to fill a tub with water without plugging the drain.

Desperation, psychological defeat, and social ostracism lead us to the dark side of life. Our only hope is that someone will recognize our plight and assist us in identifying the culprit foods.

Encouraged to Eat

Contrary to popular thought, overweight is not the result of lack of willpower. Simply pushing away from the table is too easy a concept; it insults the intelligence of patient and doctor. If it were that easy, I assure you there would not be a restaurant on every busy street corner. This drive to eat and overeat is as strong a compulsion as any drug craving, modulated by chemical reactions created in the body by foods. It is big business, capitalized on by big business.

Be it the effect on serotonin levels or the stimulation of endorphin receptors, certain people experience a sincere pleasure and euphoria from eating. This sensation is so much preferred over the status quo that we aggressively seek it to avoid the pain of reality. A common behavior in middle-aged patients is a tendency to overeat because they are unhappy with their lives. The pain and disappointment of unfulfilled dreams and expectations is too much to bear. Often increased alcohol consumption and its empty calories precede the history of overeating in these patients. But compared to the undesirable social stigma of excessive alcohol consumption, eating is socially acceptable and even encouraged by society.

Virtually all our social gatherings—from board meetings to celebrating the birth of Christ—are characterized by abundant food. Maybe this reflects our heritage as humans—to break bread together is a sign of friendship. But the tradition has gotten way out of hand. The overweight individual is placed in the precarious position of either appearing to shun the celebration or becoming an out-of-control eating machine. This no-win proposition leaves most of us choosing to eat ourselves into the euphoria that lets us escape reality. Plainly put, a common cause of overweight is social circumstances that expose those suffering from overweight to the public humiliation of succumbing to addiction. This cruel and irresponsible enticement to food is imposed daily on overweight people.

The Yeast Beast Doth Have Me

Other underlying causes of overweight are more physiological. For example, Jan, a middle-aged woman, came to my office determined to lose weight once and for all. As this was her "many-eth" time, Jan deserves credit for perseverance. In our interview we reviewed the usual eating history and cycle of weight gain and loss she had battled since childhood. Each weight loss had been followed by an equally impressive weight regain. She casually mentioned that she had been a sickly child and had many bouts of throat and ear infections. At one point Jan had been put on a variety of antibiotics for over two months. During her teenage years she put on weight and dealt from that point on with the misery of being overweight. When asked, she told of many bouts with vaginal "yeast" infections, even routinely using vaginal suppositories during her menstrual period in an effort to prevent the relentless infections that followed her cycle. Eventually marriage and pregnancy led to a C-section, followed again by a long course of antibiotics due to complications.

The overwhelming evidence said Jan was suffering from *candidiasis*, an intestinal yeast infestation that can spread systemically. Sure enough, when she was specifically asked about sweet and starch cravings, she admitted she craved sweets and especially chocolates in an inhuman way but avoided them for the obvious caloric reasons. She, however, allowed herself to enjoy bread on a daily basis as well as frequent servings of frozen yogurt, baked potatoes, and rice dishes. She had used yogurt at one time to alleviate her monthly yeast infections and associated it with health.

Jan had the ALCAT Test done, which confirmed that she had a strong reaction to several foods as well as a reaction to *Candida albicans* (yeast). This positive reaction implied that the yeast itself had entered the blood at some time, which made treatment that much more imperative. We had an extended talk about a "candida diet protocol" and her need to avoid all sweets, starches, and "yeast" foods such as bread and alcohol, as well as foods to which she had tested positive on the ALCAT Test. Appetite suppressants were prescribed to enable her to stick to the restrictive diet. Jan stayed on her diet, and to make an already long story short, she recovered quite well. Her sweet cravings subsided and, after a month of treatment with an alternative protocol for *candidiasis,* she felt more energetic. Her weight dropped nicely and she resumed eating responsibly and taking vitamin and mineral supplements to strengthen her immune system. She will be followed routinely to monitor her weight and cravings.

If her sweet cravings flare up again, Jan knows how to use the protocol to treat the "yeast" and also knows that it may become necessary to treat it with medication in the future. She understands the value of the rotation diet concept (rotating foods so the same food is not eaten more than once every four days) in the prevention of food sensitivity and eats a variety of foods. Her advantage is that she now has an option: Jan knows she does not have to be fat, and she has control of her destiny.

Although the connection is not precisely understood, intestinal yeast infections and food intolerance are closely related. Identifying Jan's reactivity to yeast was crucial—offering compelling evidence that aggressive treatment with anti-fungal medications or alternative protocols while eliminating reactive foods was appropriate. As a matter of fact, successful treatment of the yeast infection may be necessary to prevent additional food intolerance from developing.

Out with the Good and In with the Bad

With the advent of abundant antibiotics, we may be unaware of the price we pay. Many antibiotics have a devastating effect on the good bacteria in our intestine—bacteria necessary for the complete digestion of food. If these bacteria are eliminated by a prolonged round of antibiotics, the small intestine is fertile ground for the colonization of yeast. Commonly found in the throat and digestive system of healthy humans, these yeast only become a problem when the immune system is compromised. When not controlled by our immune system, these yeast reproduce rapidly and set up shop in the lining of the intestine. Once established, they can be very hard to eradicate. An estimated 25 million Americans suffer from chronic *candidiasis.*

Opportunistic Menace

The yeast itself is normally a benign casual "passerby" in the digestive tract. From the mouth and esophagus to the colon, yeast may be commonly found in healthy people. As with so many infections of the body, everything is okay until it isn't. That is, as long as the body defenses are intact and functioning properly, these casual occupants of the digestive tract are no more threatening than the food digesting therein. However, in the event that the immune system is suppressed, these opportunistic organisms quickly take advantage of the ideal conditions afforded by the intestinal tract. They attach to the lining of the intestine and easily tap into the rich blood supply. Surviving on the sugar and starches, which they ferment to use, they grow and reproduce through spores and through asexual propagation (breaking off of pieces). This dual method of reproduction enables them to propagate in different areas of the intestine by simply breaking apart and reestablishing themselves at a more favorable site.

The chronic nature of symptoms associated with food intolerance may be so insidious and subtle as to be accepted as "normal."

As the yeast population increases, so do the patient's symptoms. Physical invasion of the intestine lining, along with inflammation associated with the attachment of foreign bodies, prevents the intestinal mucosa from absorbing nutrients as usual. Additionally, because the yeast greedily extract nutrients they need for survival, the human host gets less. The immune system cells in the lining of the intestine eventually (remember, it was suppressed) respond and find themselves in a real "David and Goliath" predicament. At the same time, the lining of the intestine, now compromised by this parasite, doesn't function in its usual selective way. Larger-than-normal size particles of food may be absorbed into the bloodstream through the intestinal lining that's inflamed or irritated by the yeast.

This is, in effect, the second alarm turned in to the immune system. It now has to deal with these abnormal "foreign" particles of food as well as continue to attack the yeast. Before long the combination of continuous demand and decreasing nutritional absorption limit the ability of the immune system to function. In an all-out survival war against the yeast and food, the immune system begins to confiscate nutrients from other tissues to carry out its duties. Now fighting the war with a shrinking army, the immune system is unable to carry on its routine surveillance. Frequent viral or bacterial infections may result.

Let's stop a minute and see where we are. The human in question may well present this complaint to her physician: "I feel like I'm falling apart." Over a period of time the patient has changed from a healthy, well-functioning individual to one plagued by a multitude of miseries with no obvious cause or connection. Let us examine the events and substantiate the symptoms.

Yeast infection = craving sweets, starchy foods

Yeast infection = fatigue due to under-nutrition due to poor absorption

Yeast infection = immune system is compromised, in disarray, ineffective

Yeast infection = constipation or diarrhea, worsening absorption, allowing yeast to proliferate

Yeast infection = the integrity of the intestinal lining is compromised, allowing abnormal size particles of food to enter the bloodstream. Also, particles of yeast may enter the bloodstream and disseminate to other tissues

Yeast infection = disseminated yeast may compromise other organ systems, increasing demands on immune system. At some point endocrine organs may begin to malfunction, resulting in signs of autoimmune disease. The thyroid, the pancreas, adrenals, and the gonads are affected. Weight gain reaches logarithmic growth, fueled by the sugar and starch cravings. Insulin production cannot keep up and insulin resistance results from poor-quality insulin. Fat storage intensifies due to large amounts of sugar and insulin

Then come food sensitivities . . .

Food sensitivities = repeated exposure to food demands response of compromised immune system

Food sensitivities = increased stress on the immune system may result in other organ malfunction due to autoimmune disease

Food sensitivities = various symptoms develop depending on response of immune system to food. Sinus drainage, arthritis, irritable bowel, migraines, attention-deficit disorder, skin rashes, eczema, depression

Food sensitivities = intensified cravings, now for the serotonin or endorphin effect needed by the brain to tolerate the stress of total disintegration of orderly organ function. Depression may intensify from the feelings of helplessness

At this point, assuming nothing has been done to alleviate this rapid deterioration of the immune system, other body organs begin to malfunction. These events may cause rapid aging. Often patients relate that they are "just getting older" to justify the symptoms of food sensitivities. Like the proverbial toppling dominoes, the body begins to malfunction in a systematic fashion. Seemingly out of control, the reaction is actually the logical, predictable sequence of events resulting from a failure to treat the problem.

Granted, the above may represent a worse-case scenario. But even if the system achieves a plateau at some point in the progression, the result is a less-than-healthy body forever destined to depend on the medical community for relief of isolated symptoms. Treating the isolated symptoms as they appear prolongs the disease. Treating the yeast and food intolerance is the cure.

Eating Has Its Limits

Many overweight patients simply love to eat. Not necessarily craving any particular food, they just don't stop eating until there is no more food. These patients assume that their digestive system simply digests everything they eat. Without regard for the fact that sensitive digestive enzymes must be made by the body ahead of time and are actually in limited supply, these people only stop eating when signaled by empty plates (theirs and those of the people sitting on either side). In these individuals food intolerance seems like a contradiction; the casual observer might think they tolerate food unusually well. In fact, these patients commonly test highly reactive to a number of foods.

These obsessive eaters enter the familiar downward spiral of health as huge excesses of food overwhelm their digestive enzymes. This results in large quantities of partially digested food entering the gut. Once in the small intestine, undigested particles of food pose a great threat if they are absorbed through the intestinal wall into the bloodstream. The immune cells in the blood attack and destroy them but take their "fingerprint" as though they were an invading microbe. If it is an immune-mediated reaction, from that point on, the "allergic" reaction inten-sifies each time that food is eaten, which is frequently. The cycle is started as serotonin falls due to the allergic reaction when the reactive food is eaten. This results in further eating in an attempt to elevate the serotonin level. The process repeats itself regularly throughout the day.

Avoid overweight by eating slowly. Take at least 20 minutes to finish a meal, which should consist of appro-priate portions. Avoid buffets, all-you-can-eat specials, and allowing your mother to fill your plate for you. All these scenarios lend themselves to excessive portions. Chew and swallow food before taking another mouthful. Ask yourself: "Am I still hungry?" before each bite. If the answer is "No," stop eating. There is a huge caloric differ-ence between no longer being hungry and being "full." Preserve your digestive enzymes; you only have a limited supply; and when they run out, you are done digesting and ripe for some big-time food intolerance.

Food, the Ultimate Drug

In its broadest interpretation, food must be considered a drug. Although most of us think of drugs as potent chem-ical formulations carefully compounded by "super smart" scientists to treat disease, this mind-set intimidates us into believing that we are not smart enough to take care of our own bodies and we rush to seek professional help and their miracle drugs. In fact a large percentage of all drugs are derived from plants—food if you will (digitalis from foxglove, for example). Yes, some require extensive processing, but the fact remains that, in many cases, drugs are derived from our food. And it follows that if we can have adverse reactions to these drugs, we might also react negatively to foods. And if some drugs may have the side effects of overweight, headaches, and gastrointesti-nal distress, why do many of us find it unthinkable that food might do the same?

Call it unscientific, but this concept is so logical it need not wait for confirmation through medical school studies on thousands of patients—especially since no such study is planned. Reams of studies, however, do allude to the influence of food on various disorders. Individually, such studies are easily ignored as isolated curiosities; but when collectively viewed as food intolerance, they take on new meaning and significance.

Food is a drug with which we dose ourselves by our eating. Foods elicit specific chemical reactions in our bodies, some to our benefit and others to our detriment. Foods by definition are foreign to the body and, like all foreign objects, have the potential to be isolated and eradicated by the immune system. To minimize this event and to allow for the orderly assimilation of nutrients, our digestive enzymes are designed to break food down into its smallest components before absorption. The immune system does not react to individual amino acids, fatty acids, or short carbon chains, which represent the smallest building blocks of proteins, fats, and carbohydrates.

Likewise, the minerals and vitamins within our food are safely absorbed after proper digestion has freed them from the larger food macromolecule. Once past the immune barrier, these food components may proceed through the bloodstream to be used by the body. But in the event that food is not completely digested, the immune barrier lining in the intestine and in the bloodstream will make every effort to destroy the food as though it were a large bacteria or virus or foreign chemical. If the food macromolecule happens to pass through the intestinal lining into the bloodstream, other immune cells continue to attack and destroy it. In the process, these immune cells elicit the release of chemicals that have direct effects on the surrounding tissue. The resulting inflammation, swelling, and pain become the hall-mark of that food in the body. Thus the healthy immune response intended for an invading virus is mistakenly directed toward food that is eaten repeatedly and results in a series of symptoms.

Who Is That Masked Man?

The chronic nature of symptoms associated with food intolerance may be so insidious and subtle as to be accepted as "normal." Often patients simply accept these symptoms after repeatedly hearing from doctors that they will just have to live with them. Living with chronic symptoms is unnecessary when these symptoms are related to foods that could be eliminated. The low-grade, chronic nature of a delayed food reaction is called "masking" because it conceals the food as the perpetrator. Also, the chronic nature of the symptoms and the delay between eating the food and the appearance of symptoms makes identifying the specific offending food difficult.

Unlike tedious trial elimination diets, the ALCAT Test speeds the process of identifying the foods most likely at fault. In addition to identifying likely perpetrators, the ALCAT Test identifies "safe" foods that elicit no reaction. These foods are useful to fall back on while you conclusively identify foods responsible for your undesirable symptoms. Examples of "mask" symptoms are fatigue, chronic sinusitis, rhinitis, arthritis, depression, colitis, and attention-deficit disorder. Keep in mind that virtually any condition or symptom may be mimicked by food intolerance.

In her book *The Food Pharmacy,* Jean Carper specifically identifies the variety of drug-like effects our foods can have on us. From apples, which lower cholesterol and blood pressure to yogurt, which prevents ulcers and boosts the immune system, our foods are invaluable drugs to promote our health. And, like drugs, foods may elicit reactions other than those for which they are taken. The same apple that lowers your cholesterol may precipitate stomachaches and diarrhea days later. The yogurt may cause a rash on your arms. To embrace the potential benefits of food and fail to recognize that food may also cause many of our ills by virtue of its chemistry is closed-minded and unscientific.

To Be or Not to Be . . . Sick

Jean Carper and her experts predict that "eating in the future will increasingly be a therapeutic experience" and "people will come to depend more on foods and less on drugs to preserve health." This future experience is happening now as everyday people identify the foods that prevent them from living life to the fullest. Our future good health and happiness depends on our keen awareness of foods that keep us well and those that make us sick enough to need drugs.

According to Dr. David Satcher, director of the Centers for Disease Control and Prevention, it is unacceptable that as a nation, "We only spend 1% of our health care budget on prevention. We tend to be crisis oriented when it comes to health." We deserve more than a food pyramid of vague suggestions to stay healthy. Our schoolchildren deserve a comprehensive curriculum so they can learn that foods can help them as well as cause their miseries. Just as they are protected from tobacco, our children should be protected from sugars and processed foods that have been stripped of nutritional value.

Because these sugars and processed grains can predispose us to food intolerance, they should be avoided. They have minimal if any nutritional value, as processing removes valuable vitamins and minerals and adds sugar in amounts toxic to the brain and immune system. Separated from their naturally valuable, healthy constituents, these simple carbohydrates now only serve to derail our efficient insulin balance, resulting in a frantic storage of fat. Unfortunately the revered food pyramid does not differentiate between whole grains and processed grains, or between fresh, frozen, and canned vegetables. And the differences nutritionally between these can be vast. To clarify our unenviable situation, two of the largest industries in this country are the fast-food industry and the health-care industry. And we pass from one to the other in assembly-line monotony.

A Drug by Any Other Name

Louise arrived at her doctor's office after local news coverage of the ALCAT Test. She was 75 pounds overweight. The victim of irritable bowel syndrome for several years, she had given up taking steroid medication because it caused her to swell up so badly. She was so fatigued she often chose not to get out of bed until after noon and even then did so laboriously. Chronic sinus congestion and drainage, migraine headaches and depression—all previously diagnosed and treated symptomatically—continually plagued her.

Despite her lack of confidence in the medical system, she felt sure that foods were her problem after she heard the newscast. Like many patients, she had already made her own diagnosis. She was food intolerant but didn't know how to go about determining which foods bothered her. After the doctor heard her story and reviewed her dietary history, she was given the ALCAT Test. Before she left the office she was given instructions to avoid all "wheats and sweets" until the test results were in. Two days later she called the office to report she was feeling much better and her fatigue had disappeared. Her test results showed that she was sensitive to eggs, beef, wheat, soy, olives, and peanuts (among other foods).

Now, more convinced than ever, she began a full elimination diet in earnest. Within two weeks, every one of her symptoms had resolved with the exception of the extreme dryness of the skin on her hands. She wanted to know how long before her excess weight would come off. She was told that this would take a little longer, while she made some healthy changes in her eating habits and avoided her reactive foods.

For the first time in her adult memory, Louise was not controlled by food, bothered by a plethora of miseries leading her to overeat. She had become an exuberant schoolgirl in contrast to the defeated soul who had wandered into the office to ask about the blood test mentioned on the news. For Louise, food was a drug—a drug that precipitated bowel cramping, sinus congestion, overweight, migraine headaches, and demoralizing fatigue. Food was a drug she was willing to use with caution to avoid its devastating side effects.

CHAPTER 6

Yo-Yo Dieting

M any misconceptions about weight loss perpetuate the very problem they purport to solve. Diet medications offer temporary appetite suppression that returns with a vengeance when the drugs are stopped. Failure to take into consideration the interrelationship of food intolerance, insulin, serotonin, and thyroid leads to many confusing and unsuccessful weight-loss plans—and to what is often called "yo-yo dieting."

Yo-yo dieting has been around for a long time, but within the last 20 years it has reached national pastime proportions, probably through the popular use of appetite suppressants to speed weight loss. As their weight started going up and down faster, the descriptive term "yo-yo" captured the fancy of frustrated dieters.

"At least," they felt, "there is a name for what happens to me." Actually, it wasn't happening *to* them but *for* them. Their bodies began to rapidly conserve energy when food was scarce and rapidly store energy when food was plentiful. "Yo-yoing" characterizes a predictable biologic response. In many cases, when undiscovered food sensitivities are present, the culprit food is never completely eliminated as a reactive stimulus. Upon discontinuing medications, dieters resume previous eating habits, often including reactive foods on a regular basis. Because the documented blood reaction to intolerant food results in a decrease in serotonin levels, dieters compensate by eating serotonin-enhancing foods. Most foods that stimulate the production of serotonin also increase insulin production, which results in several things happening in your body:

1. Blood sugar will eventually drop. When it drops below a predetermined level, you will get hungry or pass out.

2. Your fat cells will open wide and store fat voraciously since you are obviously using blood sugar for energy and don't need the fat for energy.

3. Your fat cells will not release fat into your bloodstream to be used for energy because the glucose in your blood is a preferred energy source when it is available.

4. Production of eicosanoids (prostaglandins that are inflammatory mediators), which produce allergic symptoms.

None of these events are particularly good news if you are trying to lose weight. So, if we accept that the release of insulin is counterproductive to weight loss, let's identify those substances that stimulate the release of insulin into the bloodstream. Obviously, sugar in all its forms and permutations (look for items such as sucrose, fructose, dextrose, lactose, and galactose on food-ingredient labels) stimulates insulin production. It's complicated to avoid just sugars!

Well, get ready for this: Refined grains may actually raise your insulin level higher and faster than sugar. If you think this includes bread, cereal, bagels, white flour (and anything made from it), rolls, muffins, pastries, and pasta, you are right. In addition, high-sugar fruits may cause your insulin level to rise. Even the sweet taste of aspartame in your mouth causes your pancreas to start producing insulin. A large study by the American Cancer Society a few years ago yielded surprising results that received little attention. This study was to evaluate aspartame as a cancer risk. Although the carcinogenic effect of aspartame was inconclusive, the researchers noticed a curiosity among the participants ingesting aspartame-sweetened sodas on a regular basis. These subjects gained more weight than did those who drank sugar-sweetened sodas on a regular basis.

When the researchers studied this particular aspect in more detail, they learned that aspartame promotes a significant rise in insulin an hour or two later. Terrific, you think, now you have really faked out your body; you have all this insulin floating around with no sugar for it to work on. Remember what happens when you have low blood sugar (see item 1 above). That's right—you get hungry. Welcome to the merry-go-round! Now eat some sweet treat because you faithfully drank a diet drink to avoid the calories. Wait a minute—factor in the stress of juggling family, job, finances, relationships, and healthy eating. In a blink of an eye you realize that while the media had you so afraid of yo-yoing, you had actually become a one-person circus act. You are yo-yoing, juggling—and ballooning—on the merry-go-round.

It's no wonder we are confused about losing weight; even the diet food staples—pasta and diet sodas—are keeping us fat. It's as though someone gave us rules to the wrong game. Where does the madness end?

It ends with your reading books like this one and sifting through all the advertising hype. Get off the merry-go-round, put your yo-yo in your pocket, and practice juggling just two items at a time before throwing everything into the air at once. Go back to basics: drink filtered water and eat basic foods—vegetables, fruits, and meats. Shun the fancy gourmet knock-off that slathers the food with sugar and fat, freezes it, then boasts that it tastes good and is good for you. Get smart, buy a steamer and cook up a batch of fresh veggies. Relinquish sugars and refined grains to control your weight. If you think you may suffer from food sensitivities, intestinal *candidiasis,* or subclinical hypothyroidism, see a physician who will help you decide the best way to diagnose and treat these problems.

Yo-yo dieting has been around for a long time, but within the last 20 years it has reached national pastime proportions, probably through the popular use of appetite suppressants to speed weight loss.

If the stress of everyday life is contributing to your weight gain, see a physician who recognizes and promotes stress management and lifestyle adjustment programs as a valuable part of weight control. The point is, don't rush out and take appetite suppressants, herbs, or

90-day wonder cures for weight loss. Understand that something *is* wrong and it *can* be treated rather then covered.

Who Came Up with This Food Pyramid?

It is interesting that the official USDA food pyramid recommends a large sampling of grains and fruit each day. This pyramid may represent a way to assure adequate nutrient intake in the form of vitamins and minerals, but it certainly is no way to lose weight. As noted by Barry Sears in his book *The Zone,* the food pyramid closely resembles the proportions of fat, protein, and carbohydrates fed to cattle in feedlots to fatten them for slaughter. I suggest you rethink the food pyramid. If it fattens cattle so well, why would it make us thinner? Observe that "food pyramid" Americans aren't getting thinner; they are getting fatter. And that's not just a coincidence.

Processed Foods:
Are All Carbohydrates Created Equal?

Grains are nutritionally great for you—when they are whole-grain products and only when you are not sensitive to them. Whole-grain foods are not rare; they are just rarely eaten. Most grains we eat in this country have been so highly processed and adulterated that one might safely conclude their only value lies in name recognition for advertising. Overusing and overeating processed foods such as highly refined grains predisposes us to developing food sensitivities. Much is missing from this nutritionally dead food. Regardless of how much man-made nutrient is put back in after processing, the food has changed from and cannot substitute for the natural form.

But no matter how nutritionally worthless the processed food may be to the body, it can still stimulate the digestive system. Your digestive system doesn't realize you haven't the sense to avoid worthless food; it trusts that you intentionally ate this high-starch, high-sugar, and high-fat meal for a good reason. After all, you are the one with the brain.

At the expense of untold quantities of digestive enzymes, your digestive system scrounges every available nutrient from this barren wasteland, void of vitamins and minerals, called processed food. Foraging, as it will, the body is able to glean carbohydrates, fats, and a few proteins from this synthetic food. Even the man-made vitamins that "fortify" it may defy identification and use by the body. Since all the useful enzymes were removed during processing, your body must enzymatically finance this digestive venture. But, to avoid being entirely pessimistic, your pancreas responds admirably to the rise in blood sugar brought on by the processed carbohydrate that has no other nutritional value. As a result, all that nutritionally worthless fat that had been added to the processed grain to make it palatable now has set up permanent residence on your hips, thighs, and buttocks. (Maybe *that's* why they call it a food pyramid! If we eat what they tell us to, we will resemble a pyramid!)

So despite all the hope your digestive system puts into processing each meal, many meals are simply bad investments. All in all, the body must use up enzymes and hormones that are more valuable than the little nutrient available in the food.

Medications and Weight Loss: How Long Can This Go On?

Prescription medications for weight loss have become a lucrative profit center for large pharmaceutical companies.

The basic deficiency of current weight-loss medications lies in the fact that they are explicitly intended for the relief of symptoms (hunger). The treatment of overweight should not be confused with the treatment of hunger, which is what prescribing medicine is about. Although a common symptom of overweight patients, hunger is by no means the underlying cause of their overweight. Inappropriate hunger doesn't just happen; chemical changes in the body result in hunger. Resolving the symptom without diligent investigation as to the underlying cause is tantamount to teasing the patient into thinking their disease is cured. Once the medications are no longer prescribed, the unresolved or unidentified etiology of the overweight re-emerges, resulting in weight regain.

The good news is that when your reactive foods are eliminated, your problem with overweight slowly disappears.

All current medications are indicated only for relatively short periods of time. Since most studies are only done for limited periods, the medication is approved for only that time frame. If in that period of time a reasonable cause and treatment has not been established for the overweight problem, the patient would seem to be out of luck. It would be up to the discretion of the physician to extend treatment past the time approved.

This would be similar to treating the diabetic patient with insulin for the symptom of high blood sugar. If we removed the insulin as soon as the blood sugar values returned to normal, the patient would surely begin showing symptoms of high blood sugar in short order. Unless a specific remedy to renew the pancreas's ability to produce insulin is instituted, the underlying disease is not cured and treatment must continue. No one has become overweight due to a deficiency of appetite suppressant in the blood; therefore, it stands to reason that appetite suppressant should only be used with the intention of giving symptomatic relief while the true disease is investigated and treated.

Am I Really Hungry?

Granted, hunger is a contributing factor to the development of overweight. More important to the cure of overweight is the underlying drive to eat, which the patient interprets as hunger. Why do some people feel "hungry" at inappropriate times? First, I believe our discussion will benefit from a technically correct definition. "Hunger" as defined by *Webster's* dictionary is "a strong desire or need for food." In the overweight patient, "need" and "desire" for food are two very different feelings. Need implies supplying nutrient required to sustain life. Desire for food, on the other hand, implies satisfaction of a wish, a dream, a pleasure if you will. Satisfying the *need* for food would seem to carry little risk of incidental excess calories as nutritional deficiencies of the body are satisfied, but satisfying the *desire* for food carries the risks of reckless abandon as one eats to satisfy a much more ephemeral calling. Without regard for nutrients, one may consume food to ease the pain of chemical imbalances created by mental, psychological, or physiological stress. Incredible sums of unneeded calories may be consumed to alleviate stress-induced low serotonin levels, or to satiate proliferating yeast.

Nonetheless, appetite suppressants relieve hunger defined as the *desire* or *need* for food. Now if you were to take appetite suppressants to enable you to evaluate and select wise food choices that minimize unnecessary caloric intake and maximize nutrient intake, you will eliminate the incidental calories by eating needed food. If you were to take appetite suppressants to indiscriminately reduce the amount of food you eat, you may well precipitate nutrient deficiencies in your body. These in turn will result in hunger defined as the need for nutrient. A vicious cycle of gross proportions ensues.

How Should I Eat?

Appetite suppressants should be used only to allow individuals to make wise food choices, never to simply eat less food. Anyone taking appetite suppressants should seek professional guidance for proper nutrition. To assume that the overweight patient will make wise food choices because he isn't hungry is like assuming that an addict will write a master's thesis because he's gotten his drug fix. In both cases, the relief of physiologic symptoms does not make up for lack of education.

The overweight person must be taught how to properly nourish his body. To simply praise and rave over the consumption of fewer calories with no attention to life-giving nutrients is naive. A general understanding of the nutritional needs of your own body, including its food sensitivities, is imperative. You should also have a general understanding of various foods and their benefits and potential risks. You must then learn how to deal appropriately with the emotional stresses that result in your inappropriate eating.

Without intense remedial education in these areas, dieters are likely to eat less food only for a period to satisfy a short-term goal. Weight regain is expected and predictable in those who don't know how *not* to gain weight. Using appetite suppressants without making a diligent effort to determine the underlying cause of your overweight and without seeking the knowledge you need to correct your deficiencies is an injustice. Having said that, let it be understood that any medically supervised weight-control program is a partnership. It is incumbent on both partners to do their fair share. Even the best intentions of the medical professional cannot impose weight loss on an individual unwilling to make changes in eating behavior or lifestyle.

Some of the more common appetite suppressants are described below. This list is meant only to educate the reader as to some interesting attributes of each drug. Readers desiring a more in-depth understanding can refer to the *1998 Physicians' Desk Reference* or to the manufacturers' informational literature.

Phentermine Hydrochloride A sympathomimetic amine, similar in pharmacologic action to the amphetamines. Extensively studied for its anorexic properties, Phentermine is commonly prescribed as an appetite suppressant. According to the *1998 Physicians' Desk Reference,* "Adult obese subjects instructed in dietary management and treated with 'anorectic' drugs, lose more weight on the average than those treated with placebo and diet, as determined in relatively short-termed clinical trials. The magnitude of increased weight loss of drug-treated patients over placebo-treated patients is only a fraction of a pound a week."

Adverse Reactions: Possible untoward side effects of this class of drugs include palpitations, tachycardia, headache, dry mouth, dizziness and impotence, among others.

Attributes: Phentermine has been used for many years. When prescribed under monitored conditions, it is relatively safe when compared to its amphetamine cousins for control of appetite. It is available in a variety of dosage forms, which allows individualization of dosing; also available in resin, or extended-release form.

Drawbacks: Not indicated for use during pregnancy. Phentermine may give a false sense of security in control of hunger, discouraging patients from seeking out the underlying cause of their overweight. Contraindicated in a number of medical conditions, it is indicated only as a short-term (a few weeks) adjunct to weight reduction. Some brands of Phentermine include sugar, corn starch, and lactose in their preparations, which may pose a dilemma for food intolerant patients needing to eliminate these foods.

Phendimetrazine Tartrate Another sympathomimetic amine, Phendimetrazine embraces the same limitations as Phentermine above. Tolerance to the anorectic (appetite suppressant) effects usually develops in a few weeks.

Sibutramine This medication is the latest appetite control medication to be approved by the FDA. Its primary mechanism of action is to inhibit the re-uptake of serotonin, epinephrine, and dopamine in the brain. Much controversy surrounded its release. Apparently some researchers question its safety.

Attributes: Sibutramine offers appetite control through central nervous system effects on serotonin, dopamine, and epinephrine. It is taken once daily. It should not interfere with driving a car or machinery.

Drawbacks: Sibutramine may significantly raise blood pressure and pulse rates in some patients. Close monitoring is necessary throughout treatment. Many medications cannot be used while taking Sibutramine. Numerous researchers and physicians feel that long-term safety has yet to be proven.

Diethylproprion This, too, is a sympathomimetic amine with pharmacologic qualities and cautions as listed above for Phentermine. Diethylproprion has been around for a long time and is often used as a secondary appetite suppressant when resistance develops to Phentermine or Phendimetrazine.

Attributes: Convenient dosage forms in both immediate-release and timed-release formulations.

Drawbacks: There have been reports of psychological dependency on diethylproprion. Caution should be used when prescribing for patients with symptomatic cardiovascular disease or epilepsy. Contraindicated in pregnant women and nursing mothers. All of the sympathomimetic amines have possible side effects of irritability, insomnia, impotence, tachycardia, and palpitations.

FDA approval of appetite suppressants becomes almost a moot point when one realizes the inherent risks of any medication. In the Summer 1995 edition of *Health & Wellness Today,* Dr. Julian Whitaker states: "FDA approved drugs kill 140,000 people per year! That's seven times more than die from heroin, crack and all other illegal drugs put together!"

Taking appetite suppressants, fat binders, or metabolism enhancers without an overall program of food-sensitivity testing, lifestyle modification, education, stress therapy, or diagnosis of the underlying cause of the overweight is like getting in a taxi, starting the meter, and going nowhere. You will pay a lot of money to end up exactly where you started. There are no shortcuts in the treatment of overweight just as there are none in the treatment of diabetes, cancer, or congestive heart failure.

Fingerprinting Your Foods

As you repeatedly eat and overeat processed food, you may eventually exceed the capabilities of your digestive enzymes. This results in undigested or partially digested food in the intestine. The area of the intestine where absorption takes place is beyond the point at which digestion takes place. If undigested or partially digested food continues through the intestine, it is more likely to be absorbed as large food particles rather than the beneficial amino acids, fatty acids, and short carbon chains that can be used from the bloodstream with little modification.

Normally the wall of the intestine is highly selective about the size of particles it will absorb. However, if the wall of the gut is inflamed by viral infection, allergic response to food, *candida* yeast infestation, pregnancy, or any of a multitude of causes, it may absorb larger-than-normal-size food particles.

Once this larger particle of food has made it through the intestinal lining, it is for all practical purposes in the blood vessel. Here it comes under the close scrutiny of specialized immune system cells, whose job is to patrol the bloodstream watching for potential troublemakers. As these cells chemically identify the food particle, they also send off chemical signals that attract more immune system cells to the area. Eventually the food particle is neutralized and disassembled into its smallest chemical units which, interestingly, is the exact process that the digestive enzymes should have performed in the stomach and intestine.

Just as many car accidents could be avoided by people driving slower and paying more attention, so could people avoid many food sensitivities by eating slower and paying more attention to food choices. As you see, the body has set up an excellent backup system to prevent large unidentified particles from roaming around the bloodstream, whether they are viruses, bacteria, or food. And as it does with viruses and bacteria, the immune system memorizes the chemical fingerprint of the food. In the future, anytime it sees that "fingerprint" again, it will attack it with even greater vigor as a repeated "threat" to the body.

Familiarity Leads to Contempt

Let's just say that the food to which you have now become sensitive (when you eat it, your immune system reacts to it in an ever-increasing intensity) happens to be one you eat every day. Perhaps it's milk, or wheat, or corn. Over a period of time the violent immune reaction to the food will result in more and more local tissue response in an attempt to isolate this invader from the rest of the body. As this "allergic reaction" spreads to surrounding tissues, the symptoms you have will represent the swelling and diminished function of body organ systems. When the lining of your colon swells up because of a food you ate, abdominal cramps and diarrhea may fill your day. If the food stimulates a response in the stomach, expect the fires of "acid reflux" to flare. If the allergic food makes it into your bloodstream, you may experience the misery of anything from "sinus congestion" to migraine headaches to skin rashes and "arthritis." This great "mockingbird of disease" may have you taking a fistful of different medications and thinking that you "are falling apart." Until you consider food as a cause of your misery, you may finance many cars and swimming pools for conventional medical practitioners.

So now you have a clearer picture of the mechanism by which indigestion, irritable bowel, colitis, and malabsorption are related to food sensitivities. Over a period of time, the immune response may signal a perpetual state of high alert as you continue to eat the same foods. Soon enough the immune system's demands for nutrients will exceed your digestive system's now-compromised ability to process and absorb nutrients.

Food Sensitivities, the Immune System, and the Thyroid

Once you have a food sensitivity, your immune system goes into hyper-drive to protect you from this persistent "invader." Over time, whether from malnutrition or just plain overactivity, your immune system goes a little haywire. It gets confused and misfires, and may even attack body parts because it can no longer distinguish between good and bad cells. This is bad enough when it results in arthritis (a common symptom associated with food sensitivities), but gets serious when it involves the thyroid.

Autoimmune destruction of the thyroid leads to decreased production of thyroid hormone. Autoimmune disease and subsequent hypothyroidism is sometimes discovered following a pregnancy. Curiously, food intolerance commonly develops during pregnancy as well. Researchers are investigating the effect of subclinical hypothyroidism on the other endocrine organs. This hypothyroidism may be the result of autoimmune destruction of part of the thyroid gland and may result in elevated insulin levels, elevated cholesterol, ovarian hormone dysfunction, depression, and weight gain due to lowered basal metabolic rate (the thyroid determines metabolic rate).

A prominent researcher in this field, Dr. Broda Barnes, gives an excellent review in his book *Hypothyroidism: The Unsuspected Illness.* To condense the excellent treatment he gives this disease process in his book would be presumptuous. Suffice it to say that the thyroid blood tests commonly used today may not give a true picture of your thyroid function. If you are cold all the time; have a high cholesterol level; suffer from menstrual irregularities, depression, hypertension, fatigue, and unexplained overweight, you would be well served by reading the book. Take it along as you seek a doctor who will treat you as a person rather than a blood test. There is no greater insult than to hear that because the blood test is normal, nothing is wrong; it's all in your mind. It makes one want to ask, "Well, doctor, if nothing is wrong, will you ask the blood test why I keep getting fatter?"

There is a distinct relationship between food sensitivities, intestinal *candidiasis,* and hypothyroidism. The symptoms of each are similar and overlapping. The conditions can and should be treated separately, but until the food sensitivities are treated, nagging symptoms will persist.

So, the bottom line is this: How do food sensitivities keep you fat? The exact mechanism may never be known, but the smoking gun seems to be in the hand of the thyroid gland at present. The good news is that when your reactive foods are eliminated, your problem with overweight slowly disappears. This would seem consistent with a thyroid mediated effect in that it takes time for the thyroid to recover.

An inflammatory response is documented in the bloodstream following the absorption of a reactive food. Presumably this inflammatory or "allergic reaction" has the potential to damage local organs and tissues if the reaction is prolonged or intense enough. Certainly this reaction consumes large amounts of nutrients and energy as the immune network of the body struggles to protect us from our food.

With time the immune system becomes more frantic as it senses it is not able to control the invading organism (food). Decreasing nutritional absorption, increasing demands on immune cells, and limitations imposed on the immune system by stress hormones result in anarchy in the immune network. Much like soldiers revolting against tyranny, the immune system begins to attack the endocrine organs, as well as other body tissues. Of the organs most susceptible and sensitive to "autoimmune" disease, the thyroid, the pancreas, and the ovaries appear to have a major influence on our weight. Let's not get bogged down in the philosophical one-upmanship that is the hallmark of conventional "ego-medicine." The fact is that many women experience thyroiditis (thyroid inflammation) following pregnancy, which may later result in a lowering of thyroid function. We also know that food sensitivities can result in autoimmune destruction of organs and that pregnancy is a common time to develop food sensitivities.

This probably results from disturbances of gastrointestinal function and absorption related to hormonal changes associated with pregnancy. Not only does the thyroid control the body's metabolic rate through the hormones it secretes, but it also affects the other endocrine organs and the hormones they secrete as well. For example, as thyroid hormone levels drop, the effect on the pancreas is to increase insulin secretion and the effect on the liver is to increase cholesterol levels and stimulate the conversion of carbohydrates to fat for storage.

Changes in thyroid hormone levels may have seemingly irrational effects on ovarian hormone production. These fluctuating hormone levels result in menstrual irregularities and pre-menopausal symptoms that often defy treatment. Treating these symptoms is difficult because it is like trying to hit a moving target as the hormone levels fluctuate wildly in response to erratic thyroid hormone levels from the sick or failing thyroid. Some degree of control is possible if one does not depend on the usual thyroid blood tests as the unequivocal measure of thyroid hormone activity at the cellular level.

Body Temperature Tells the Thyroid Story

The current blood tests we have for evaluating thyroid function are much better screening tests than those available in the past. But using a screening test to evaluate the true effect of thyroid hormone on its end organ cells does not make good sense. As we all know, quality and quantity are very different measurements and must not be confused. At this point one is not questioning whether a certain level of hormone is available in the blood or not. We need to know whether the level of thyroid hormone in the blood is adequately stimulating the appropriate cells and adequately maintaining an appropriate metabolic rate.

One simple way to evaluate clinically the effect of thyroid hormone is to monitor a patient's basal body temperature. For all practical purposes (barring fever, illness, or effects of drugs), the basal body temperature reflects the metabolic activity and clinically correlates closely with thyroid hormone function.

The first mistake is trying to treat symptoms to effect a cure. Symptoms should be used to help identify the problem; treatment should be directed at solving the problem. Symptoms are alleviated at the discretion of a compassionate physician. Treatment, on the other hand, is a commitment, a partnership, a goal-oriented effort to improve quality of life through the correction of inborn or self-induced deficiencies in body functions. The point is that the job is simply not done until the cause of the symptoms is corrected.

If you took your car to a mechanic because it was making a noise and he told you to turn the radio up and the noise would go away, I doubt you would feel confident that your problem had been solved. But how many of us leave our doctor's office with medicine to cover up the signs of our diseases of overweight, hypertension, diabetes, and menstrual irregularities? Like the figurative ostrich sticking his head in the sand, we believe that if we don't see a problem, it doesn't exist. Well, if you don't look for a problem, you will never see it. The "body mechanics" who identify and eliminate food sensitivity offer the limitless rewards of a fully functional reconditioned body with a renewed factory-serviced warranty.

Most importantly, keep in mind that even after you have your computer serviced, you still must decide which programs to load to serve your needs best. You may still have work to do regarding the various chronic conditions influenced by food sensitivities. At least you have "fixed the computer" by eliminating your reactive foods. Thyroid, insulin, and serotonin will be freed from the influence of food intolerance, and eating and exercising right will show further results in weight loss.

CHAPTER 7

Food Intolerance: The Missed Diagnosis

Virtually every human who comes to recognize food sensitivities as the source of their physical ailments feels as though their story is unique and incredible. We are so indoctrinated that foods cannot be the cause of our misery that we feel as though we are a medical wonder. In fact, we may be nothing more than the misinformed majority.

My Story

I can't say the exact day it happened, but I can tell you it felt like the floor disappeared from under me. The day I realized that food intolerance was responsible for my obesity, my attitude toward medicine changed. For almost 20 years as a physician, I had pretty much accepted the conventional mind-set. I treated symptoms and treated them well, sometimes over and over again in the same patient. Nonetheless my patients' gratitude satisfied my ego as they acknowledged me as a good and caring physician. Despite my caring demeanor, I had an intense dread of treating overweight patients. I was frustrated that these patients could not understand—their overweight interfered with my treatment.

Actually I was frustrated by my inability to treat their overweight successfully, because what I knew about treating obesity was woefully inadequate. Because it seemed only a matter of willpower to push away from the table, I chastised them for not simply eating less. I now apologize to all these patients. You were ill and, because I didn't know how to help you, I passed the blame. I know now that you had no more control over your eating than the diabetic has over his pancreas.

My professional existence at the time was based on my extensive knowledge (memorizing) of chemical concoctions. These relieved symptoms until the body could cure itself. In my later practice years I depended entirely on the use of chemicals as an anesthesiologist. Even in this profession I dreaded the overweight patient for the increased risks imposed. Obesity, an illness for which I had not learned a treatment, was an affront to my skill as a doctor.

Not until I caught the disease and faced the monster myself did I appreciate the devastating effect obesity has on the quality of life.

My own health began to deteriorate the year my daughter was born and my wife was diagnosed with breast cancer. My wife died a year and a half after our daughter's birth. Then circumstances beyond my control forced me to seek other job opportunities. Meanwhile, my health continued to deteriorate over the years as my weight increased steadily through another marriage and a divorce. I was disgusted by my weight—245 pounds on a 5'9" frame. Job stress increased, and I became unable to adequately care for my eight-year-old daughter and fulfill my responsibilities as a medical school anesthesiology instructor. I was a mess.

Just because fitness gurus proclaim a low-calorie food "healthy" doesn't make it so.

At the time of my divorce I decided to change my life. I lost 45 pounds in a physician-supervised weight-loss program using medication. Feeling redeemed and enlightened by having trimmed down, I resigned my medical school instructor position and began the necessary studies to become board-certified in bariatric medicine the following year. I opened my own medical weight management office. My health was recovering and job stress was much reduced. Nutritional supplements and healthy eating habits were making all the difference. When I opened my own office, I had maintained my 200-pound weight for about six months. Not thin, but stabilized at a weight I found acceptable.

I first learned about food intolerance at a medical conference. Curious about the relationship of food intolerance to overweight, I had the ALCAT Test run on myself. I was about to go through the most rapid growth spurt of my professional life. I can remember shaking my head when I looked at my test results—positive to corn, wheat, tomatoes, beans, peppers, and turkey among other things. It baffled me to think that these "healthy" foods could contribute to my overweight problem. Most of them had, in fact, been staples of my recent successful weight loss. Nonetheless, I made the commitment and was determined to see it through.

I attacked the elimination of corn and wheat at the same time, and soon learned that 75 percent of the packaged goods at the grocery store contain corn or corn products. Wheat, on the other hand, turned up in the ingredients of all sorts of cereals, snacks, frozen entrees, and breads. Regular trips to a local health-food store became routine. Things started to fall into place once I became a dedicated label reader. Without realizing it, I had become addicted to corn and wheat. Fortunately, there are many acceptable substitutes for wheat and corn. In fact, a whole subculture of enlightened individuals who scorn traditional grocery stores are turning instead to merchants who offer wide varieties of organic produce and alternatives to common grains.

The other vegetables and the meat to which I was sensitive were easier to avoid. I distributed the peppers, tomatoes, and beans in my robust garden that year to family and friends, and changed my eating habits. After a couple months I became pleasantly aware that my craving for sweets had disappeared. My daughter could actually make her chocolate chip cookies and not worry that they would disappear while she was at school. Most remarkably, my weight resumed its downward spiral. I became more alert and had more energy than I'd had since college. I felt alive now that fatigue was no longer part of my daily existence. It was as though the accumulation of years of digestive sediment and barnacles of malnutrition had been scraped away.

Surprisingly, after the first difficult two weeks, I don't remember any discomfort from cravings or hunger. As long as I only ate when I was hungry and avoided my reactive foods, I ate whatever I wanted and lost weight each week. That's not to say that I ate what others may have wanted me to eat, but using basic common sense in avoiding fats and sugars, I lost weight effortlessly to the 175-pound range I have maintained for over a year now. I didn't have a nutrition degree, food scale, stair stepper, Richard Simmons tape, or nasty-tasting diet-in-a-can. I really did eat what I wanted; I just didn't want a lot of the unhealthy foods as long as I avoided my reactive foods.

How Do You Know When You React to a Food?

One particular episode comes to mind. My daughter and I, late for a school function, decided to grab something fast to eat on the way. Because of my food sensitivities I was preparing most of our meals because restaurants tend to mix foods for flavor, making it unrealistic for me to eat out and stay on my elimination diet. Nevertheless, we stopped at a fast-food restaurant and, for some reason, the picture of a hot bowl of chili called to me. I'm not particularly fond of chili, but food sensitivities do funny things to your mind. It is not uncommon to crave the very food to which you are sensitive.

At any rate, halfway through the bowl of chili I thought, "This has to have tomatoes in it." In a minor panic I stopped eating. It had been two full weeks since I had eaten tomatoes. About an hour later, a half-hour into the school program, I was overwhelmed with an intense headache and fatigue. I could not force my eyes to stay open to watch the program. Thankfully we made it through the program and got home safely. (Because driver fatigue is a cause of numerous accidents, I wonder how many food-sensitivity victims fall asleep at the wheel.)

I had learned a valuable lesson to pass on to my patients. Make the commitment to eliminate the food that causes you unpleasant symptoms and you will be held to that commitment. I had reneged on my commitment by unintentionally eating tomatoes in the chili. My immune system soon recognized this almost-forgotten "invader" and attacked it in a hyper-acute response. This premature reintroduction of a reactive food after a period of elimination resulted in a rapid deployment of immune system soldier cells. These cells along with the chemical reactions they elicited in the surrounding cells brought about headache, fuzzy thinking, fatigue, and runny nose. This personal experience brought to my reality a dramatic event I had only read about.

Must I Forever Forsake My Favorite Foods?

I have since reintroduced all my reactive foods into my diet. I know I cannot eat turkey without developing fatigue, and that cooked tomatoes will give me a headache. I realize my limits, and life is good when I respect these limitations.

While classical allergy reactions are pretty much permanent, in the case of food sensitivities, remove the food for a period of time and the body often forgives and forgets. Commonly after a period of three months, reintroducing the food is worthwhile. If it elicits no immediate reaction, the food can be rotated through your diet about every four days with little likelihood that you'll become sensitive to it again.

Some foods simply aren't worth the trouble. One patient expressed this opinion when reminded that she could reintroduce corn to her diet. In encouraging her to overcome the difficulties in eliminating corn from her diet, I had vividly educated her in all the digestive vagaries and ill-effects associated with corn and corn products. Apparently I had been quite convincing. When I suggested she try corn again, she responded as though I had offered her poison, politely saying: "I don't think so."

Case Studies

The following histories of patients suffering from food intolerance gives some insight into the wide variety of chronic conditions amenable to cure by eliminating reactive foods. In the following case presentations, certain identifying characteristics have been changed to protect patient privacy. The stories, however, are true.

Chronic and Neglected

One cannot experience a more empathetic moment than while performing a physical examination on an overweight female patient with chronic sinus drainage, a diagnosis of irritable bowel syndrome, and hypothyroidism who is depressed. She evokes compassion not so much because of her individual diseases, but because she represents a neglected human contingent. This group of people has been over-treated and under-cured by conventional medicine. Instructed that they will have to live with the limitations of their "chronic disease," these patients withdraw from the spotlight of society. They survive in solitude in the shadow of their former lives.

This poor woman had been shuttled between medical specialists like a hockey puck. After each extensive exam, she was told confidently that everything checked out okay and they could find nothing wrong. Each specialist—ENT (ear, nose, and throat), endocrinologist, gastroenterologist, and psychiatrist—succeeded only in proving he or she didn't know why the woman had her symptoms. But appropriate prescription medication would take care of her discomfort. Frustrated, she turned even more frequently to her one solace—her favorite foods. Not surprisingly, her symptoms persisted, and she was led to believe she would need medication the rest of her life.

Gladys, at the age of 56, had conceded she would never lead a normal life. She was seeking help for overweight—which was ruining her life—out of desperation. Her sinus and bowel problems and depression could be covered up with medication, but her weight blatantly called attention to her despair and humiliation. She desperately wanted someone who would treat her obesity with dignity.

When asked about her weight, her desperation poured out. To the point of tears, she shook her head violently and blurted out, "I just don't know what else to do! I watch what I eat, but I just keep getting bigger." Although she was calorie-conscious and carefully avoided sugars and fats, she ate an abundance of processed carbohydrates. She had noticed that milk caused stomach pains and fatigue, so she avoided it. All Gladys's symptoms showed up on the list of common symptoms associated with food intolerance. Because of her history, we decided to perform the ALCAT Test to see whether she had other food intolerances of which she was unaware.

Years of endless defeat had led her to make her own diagnosis, one that had eluded all the specialists she had consulted. She instantly knew that her body was reacting to a food or foods. That was why no one could find anything wrong; nothing *was* wrong where they were looking. Her entire problem was hidden in her own blood vessels and in the lining of her intestine, where her cells were violently attacking food particles as though they were foreign viruses or bacteria. She could not access her fat stores for energy because of the perpetual chemical reaction that paralyzed the breakdown of her fat for energy. To have any energy at all, she had to eat more food because her vast warehouse of energy was locked. Her immune system was frazzled by poor nutrient absorption through a gut wall swollen from reaction to her food. This crippled immune system was misfiring and the autoimmune diseases of hypothyroidism and arthritis probably represented its attacking the body itself. This avalanche of disease probably began with the absorption of poorly digested food into the bloodstream from the intestine.

It is not uncommon to crave the very food to which you are sensitive.

Just because fitness gurus proclaim a low-calorie food "healthy" doesn't make it so. Each food can have a totally individual and different relationship with each person. To cure many chronic illnesses, the doctor must consider food and its potential for disease in each patient. This time-consuming and dedicated approach is beyond the scope of our current "ten-minute visit" medical system. Long forgotten are the words of Hippocrates, the father of medicine: "Let thy food be thy medicine."

Happily, Gladys underwent the ALCAT food sensitivity test, and her symptoms began to resolve quickly after her elimination diet and vitamin and mineral supplements began. Her depression lifted, her irritable bowel calmed, and her sinuses cleared quickly; she now only suffers from an occasional seasonal sinus congestion. We postponed the prescription of appetite suppressants until we saw the results of the food-elimination program: four pounds lost during the first week. She now knew which foods she could not eat.

While she remained on the food-elimination diet, she continued to lose an average of two pounds per week. After losing 21 pounds, her weight had stabilized. She now felt in control of her destiny. Although she may still make an occasional poor food selection, she makes informed choices and knows the consequences; she is finally beginning to understand and make peace with her body.

We also decided to monitor her basal body temperature to evaluate thyroid function. Over a ten-day period her basal temperature averaged 3 degrees below normal. This, along with her continuing morning fatigue, dry skin and hair, and cold intolerance suggested subclinical hypothyroidism. We reviewed the options with her and she elected to try low-dose thyroid supplementation. After two months it was hard to recognize her as the same woman who had come looking for help with her weight. She was now an alert, involved member of the human race. Her basal body temperatures were rising toward normal and her clinical thyroid blood tests remained in the normal range. With time and continued attention to avoiding her reactive foods, she may be able to decrease her thyroid medication in the future—a successful outcome considering that all she wanted in the first place was diet pills.

Fibromyalgia in a Medical Professional

A 45-year-old medical professional came to me for treatment of overweight. Very dedicated, she had successfully lost weight using medication. On her initial visit she had mentioned other physical problems, including fibromyalgia that at times was debilitating. Studies into food allergies and intolerances had revealed a possible food connection to fibromyalgia. This patient was informed about this possibility and was willing to give it a try.

She had the ALCAT Test performed. She found the results very interesting and dedicated herself to quickly eliminating her reactive foods from her diet. In short order (about two weeks), she experienced significant improvement in her condition. After a few more weeks her fibromyalgia, from which she had suffered for years, was completely resolved.

After a few months she experienced a relapse. Careful questioning revealed that she had unintentionally reintroduced some of her reactive foods. With stringent elimination of those foods, she again experienced relief of her symptoms. Through her own trial and error, she was soon able to confirm that if she ate corn in any form, her fibromyalgia returned; she also discovered that tomatoes caused her gastrointestinal discomfort. She was now in control. Even though at times she chose to eat these foods, she knew the resulting symptoms were no mystery. Knowing their cause made her symptoms less intimidating, and her ability to control their occurrence allowed her a freedom she had not known for years.

ALCAT Test Confirms Food Sensitivities

One 42-year-old male patient had been under the care of his physician for several years for overweight. He had been successful at losing 20 pounds and keeping it off. He simply went once a month to see his doctor, who gave him a prescription for Fen-Phen. Following the removal of Fenfluramine from the market, his doctor would no longer treat him for overweight.

On his first visit to a new doctor, after reviewing his history, the doctor asked if he might be interested in trying a different approach to maintaining his weight. He was open to the idea of not taking medication if he could keep his weight off without it. He had the ALCAT Test done, and the results were impressive to him. He was re-active to milk, corn, and wheat among other foods.

After discovering his reactive foods, he related that he had once passed out after eating two mouthfuls of ice cream, which contains both milk and corn. He had ap-parently had a pretty intense reaction to both and should eliminate them. Going down the list of his reactive foods, he confirmed that most were foods that he enjoyed daily while successfully losing his excess weight taking medica-tion. These foods were a time bomb waiting to explode as soon as he stopped taking medication. By eliminating these foods he would be able to avoid his historic rapid weight regain.

He was also introduced to the concept of food rota-tion so he would not eat the same foods more than once every four days. This would allow his body to process and clear the innocent mistakes made by his immune system as it continued trying to protect his body from perceived invaders. He welcomed the opportunity to stop taking medication and still keep his weight off.

Attention-Deficit Disorder and Sugar Intolerance

A 13-year-old girl was brought to the office following a news broadcast of the potential benefits of eliminating reactive foods in the treatment of ADD. At an early age she had been put on Ritalin and other medication for ADD at the recommendation of teachers and doctors. After giving her medication for a couple of years, her parents decided to stop. The little girl confirmed that the medicine made her feel "funny" and she didn't like it. She also admitted that she didn't like it when her mind wandered and she forgot to do things she was supposed to do. She said she could not help it and found it embarrassing.

She related that school was becoming more and more difficult and she had received her first "F." In addition to her ADD, she had suffered from recurrent ear infections when she was younger and had strange itchy skin rashes that would come and go. One on her right leg remained itchy and scaly. Her sinus drainage problems were a constant sniffing, coughing presence. Her eating history was loaded with sugar. Interestingly, a good bit of the sugar in her diet came with the blessing of the school that diagnosed her with ADD, resulting in years of medication. After a heart-to-heart talk with mother and daughter regarding the immediate elimination of all sugars and corn products from the girl's diet, she had the ALCAT Test done, which confirmed her intolerance to sugar and corn.

In tears, the little girl blurted out, "You mean I can never eat anything sweet?" The terror of life without sugar meant a sudden coming to terms with what, for all practical purposes, was a drug addiction to sugar. This girl's ADD was nothing more than the normal bodily response to her sugar addiction.

As a matter of principle, any school system that presumes to offer the best possible learning environment for our children cannot offer them sugar. The soft-drink machine, candy rewards, and bake sales are unhealthy for all and poison for some. Giving children sugar and asking them to learn and behave may be unrealistic.

Attention-Deficit Disorder Caused by Foods

Nine-year-old Trevor appeared with his mother in the office, exhibiting the classic symptoms of attention deficit/hyperactivity disorder. It was not necessary to do a battery of tests to confirm this. (Besides, the furniture and equipment could not have withstood a longer visit.) After discussing the possibility that food intolerance was contributing to Trevor's difficulties at school and at home, we agreed to proceed with the ALCAT Test. Trevor's mother had already noticed that some foods seemed more stimulating to Trevor than others.

Discussing food intolerance with a mother who has thought the problem through and already realizes that some foods are contributing to their child's learning difficulties is a rewarding experience. Within the last year Trevor had begun to have difficulties with grades at school. He had gone from receiving solid A's and B's to getting F's. Teachers had commented to his mother that Trevor was having a hard time concentrating and recommended testing for attention-deficit disorder and Ritalin therapy. Admirably, she resisted this easy way out and began investigating on her own. She learned that foods often contribute to ADD and hyperactivity and was determined to try this avenue before considering drugs for her child.

Trevor was reactive to a number of his favorite foods, including chocolate and cane sugar. Upon learning the results of the ALCAT Test, he exploded in a fit of crying anger when told which foods he would need to eliminate. His mother elegantly accepted the information and started the elimination diet in earnest that day. A week later Trevor and his mom returned. Smiling and relieved, Mom related that Trevor had actually finished all his homework that week and that his grades were much better. He was able to concentrate and his hyperactivity symptoms were much improved. Even Trevor expressed that he felt better and didn't like the feeling he had before.

Surgical Sniffles

A middle-aged surgeon undergoing weight management had chronic rhinitis and sinus drainage. This had caused him considerable discomfort and frequent mask changes during surgery. He was constantly clearing his throat and found it annoying. After having the ALCAT Test and beginning the elimination diet, his sinus condition and rhinitis cleared up almost immediately. The elimination of reactive foods also allowed him to continue losing weight down to his goal. Months later he continues to maintain his weight by avoiding his reactive foods. His chronic sinus drainage is now only an unpleasant memory.

Foods Can Be a Real Headache

At age 14, John had been suffering classical migraine headaches for several years. The headaches were unpredictable and had ruined a number of family outings for him. Although he avoided the usual foods routinely associated with migraine headaches, he continued to have them unpredictably. Having undergone the usual battery of tests for migraine headache, he was prescribed Imitrex to try and control the headaches after they appeared. The ALCAT Test revealed he was intolerant of a number of foods that neither he nor his family had suspected. Upon his eliminating these foods, John's headaches disappeared. He only experienced a headache when he unintentionally ate a culprit food. After this he became very conscious of avoiding his reactive foods—specifically bananas.

Tired of Fatigue

A 56-year-old grandmother called the doctor's office after the first week of elimination diet proclaiming that her fatigue was gone. After years of debilitating fatigue and gradual weight gain, she felt like a new woman. After a month on the elimination diet based on her ALCAT Test results, her sinus drainage, depression, and burning indigestion had all resolved without medication.

Bad Genes, Yeast, and Food Intolerance

A 40-year-old professional woman and mother of four teenagers came to me for weight management with a chief complaint of "bad genes." Her mother and sisters were all over 20 pounds overweight, and she only dreamed of losing her 20 extra pounds. She had most recently been on a strict 1,000-calorie, low-fat diet and had been exercising vigorously to no avail. Her favorite foods were "sweets and carbohydrates." She admitted eating very fast and had been known to consume entire packages of cookies without remorse.

After discovering her food intolerances via the ALCAT Test, she began her elimination diet with commitment. Her diet was further restricted because of a positive ALCAT Test for *candida* yeast. Using only Nystatin (anti-yeast) as medication, she lost 12 pounds in six weeks. Free of sweet cravings for the first time that she could remember, she now anticipated truly losing to near her ideal weight.

All these people were made sick from the food they ate. Likewise, they became well only after deliberately avoiding the food that caused their illness. If you have food intolerance that is making you ill, only by eliminating that food will you get well. No medication, no surgery, and no therapy will succeed until you eliminate your reactive foods.

To Test or Not to Test

One reason conventional medicine finds it difficult to accept the concept of food sensitivity is that no standard treatment protocol is available. Each patient must be seen and treated on the basis of his or her unique symptoms. Add to that the time lag of up to 72 hours before symptoms may occur, and the variables boggle the imagination and the office schedule.

Using the interminable method of rotating foods through elimination phases just to detect an improvement in symptoms taxes the perseverance and trust of the most dedicated patient. The ALCAT Test dramatically improves the process of successfully diagnosing and treating food sensitivity reactions. A simple blood test, a few days' wait, and you are ready to climb into the food-elimination saddle. After undergoing the ALCAT Test, you will enter the food elimination phase with a higher degree of confidence and expectation. You will know, with about 80 percent accuracy, the foods to which you are reactive. By yourself or with the help of a knowledgeable practitioner, you can begin eliminating your reactive foods.

It may be wise to seek a professional recommendation as to dietary alternatives and/or specific nutrient supplements, depending on how many and what types of food you need to eliminate. Experience shows that patients notice a significant improvement in various symptoms within the first month; symptoms associated with sinus, headache, and indigestion often improve within two weeks. This is a great impetus to continue the elimination.

Trying to determine my own reactive foods without the benefit of the ALCAT blood test would have been frustrating. Although the test does not pretend to be 100 percent accurate, it eliminates 80 percent of the trial and error that would otherwise be necessary. Just one episode like mine with the chili was enough. The thought of going through that repeatedly during trial-and-error elimination is distasteful (pun intended).

Additionally, the recommended rotation diet that was customized to my own food sensitivities introduced me to a variety of new foods that I still enjoy. Even with hundreds of foods available, most of us eat the same 20 foods in different combinations day after day. All of us would do well to eat a wide variety of fruits and vegetables and decrease the likelihood of developing sensitivities to a particular food that we eat regularly. Without the thorough repertoire of foods allowed and organized for me by the ALCAT Test, eliminating my reactive foods would have been difficult and boring.

Early humans probably did not have to deal with unpleasantries associated with food sensitivity because they, by default, couldn't eat foods not in season or not available to hunt. Today, with a grocery store within a few miles of most Americans, we can indulge in any type of fruit, vegetable, or meat year-round and perpetually stoke the fires of a raging food sensitivity. Science serves us well technologically, but economics prevents the wide dissemination of information that would enable us to make wise choices in our best interest.

We need to know that food sensitivities are a potentially serious problem before we will consider testing to identify and avoid them. Disseminating this preventive information would seem the responsibility of the medical system, yet medical professionals have no great incentive for doing so. After all, if we were to stop getting patients with migraine headaches, ear infections, sinus drainage, indigestion, overweight, coronary artery disease, ADD, hyperactivity, and breathing and skin problems, who will fill the waiting rooms of doctors and hospitals?

CHAPTER 8

Food Sensitivities and Overweight

The likelihood of food sensitivities in individuals who are overweight is strong, if not certain. The very nature of overweight suggests an inappropriate response to food since it is not uncommon to find overweight people who eat less food and exercise more than would be indicated by their body fat. Rather than insinuate that a person is confused about the volume of food he or she eats, medical professionals should conduct food-sensitivity testing to detect any reactive foods. By eliminating these foods, people who test positive for food sensitivities can resume a "normal" weight loss appropriate for calorie intake and exercise.

Let Them Eat Bread

A logical explanation has finally surfaced for the uncontrollable desire to eat inappropriate foods at inappropriate times. Do you crave pasta tonight because of the dinner rolls you ate yesterday? Sound wild? Yes, but wilder yet is the fact that some people who don't eat wheat regularly find themselves getting up in the middle of the night to go buy it. This addiction affliction is like any other. You crave the very substance that is destroying your body. The only differences between food and other addictions are:

- Food is legal.
- Food is socially acceptable and encouraged for its known pleasurable pharmacological effects.
- Food addiction/sensitivity produces a variety of symptoms that are treatable on a recurrent basis by your doctor.
- There is no stigma directly associated with food sensitivities (but those suffering from unpredictable bouts of migraine, sinus drainage, eczema, and irritable bowel are stigmatized).

The Heartbreak of Food Sensitivities

The emotional stress placed on those afflicted with food sensitivity is monumental. These individuals may gradually become ostracized by others due to their symptoms, which restrict their activities. This contributes to decreased self-esteem, depression, and stress.

These conditions in turn place further demands on the immune system, which is already significantly fatigued by its all-out response to normal foods. To absolve these negative personal feelings, victims often instinctively turn to relief in the form of the chemical serotonin. When present in the brain in adequate amounts, this chemical neurotransmitter can temporarily turn the world rosy. Needless to say, this quick fix fades relatively soon but is easily renewed by the carbohydrate load of a bowl of ice cream, cookies, or pasta (sort of a *fix du jour*).

In fact, those of us conscientious enough to avoid the obviously fat-building foods such as refined sugars can often achieve the same peaceful state by eating (or overeating) pasta, bread, cereal, or any number of refined "low-fat" or "no-sugar" foods. The dilemma is processed foods that enhance serotonin also stimulate other body hormones such as insulin. The end result is that the more one eats for the serotonin effect, the fatter one gets.

Sadly the serotonin effect is, in the case of food sensitivities, temporary at best. When you eat a food to which you are sensitive, you stress your body, actually creating a decrease in serotonin in the eating center of the brain, but not necessarily immediately. For example, say a person is sensitive to corn. If she eats a food sweetened with corn syrup, or even a corn chip, the immediate result may be a familiar reaction in the body resulting in increased serotonin. Concurrently, however, the food may activate the immune system, resulting in various other chemical reactions depending on the immune system response to the food.

If the cells in the intestinal lining try to control the "invader," one may experience any of various symptoms the body uses to tell us that something is wrong in our intestines. For example, you might experience swelling of the mucosa (lining of the intestine) and a slowing of motility, or constipation, or malabsorption of important nutrients that results in prolific mucous secretion as the irritated lining urges the body to wash this substance away. At this point, the urgent painful moments on the porcelain throne are legendary.

If the invading food particle is identified and attacked in the blood vessels, this may result in vasculitis, damage to the blood vessel lining. As the blood vessels desperately try to clear this chemical reaction away, they dilate, or open up. This dilatation may well lead to severe headaches as well as irritability and muscle pains. Certain foods may cause symptomatic reactions affecting the brain while others may affect the sinuses, intestines, skin, or joints. Not every individual will be affected in the same way by each reactive food, but a particular food seems to result in the same symptoms each time it is eaten by the same individual.

Immune Dictatorship

The immune system has total autonomy. If it believes something is bad, our immune system exercises its authority to call forth all the body's energies to protect it. No wonder so many of us with food sensitivities are tired! Once the immune cells have branded a food as an "invader," the food will evoke the wrath of the immune response each time it is detected in the blood, regardless of how healthy it may seem. And once a food is branded as an invader, each subsequent exposure confirms this. It is a perfect example of guilty until proven innocent. This results in an incredible amount of resources being wasted fighting an imaginary enemy. As "invader foods" continue to be eaten and absorbed, the body continues consuming body energy, vitamins, and nutrients to maintain the massive "immune army" necessary to keep the body safe from the persistent food invaders.

One a Day or Ten a Day?

Few of us are aware of the quantity of vitamins and minerals we routinely need; even the most knowledgeable don't know where they stand. With the decreased absorption and outrageous consumption of the nutrients required to maintain the increased activity of the immune system, we can easily become deficient in essential nutrients. There is some logic to the idea that as we become deficient in nutrients, the body will send us to eat. Under the stress of this continuous war going on in our bodies, what do you suppose sounds good to eat? Right—something to boost serotonin. But probably not something loaded with vitamins and minerals.

ALCAT: User Friendly

After using the ALCAT food sensitivity test extensively, one cannot help but be impressed with its accuracy and versatility. It doesn't simply measure your level of a blood constituent and leave your doctor to figure out what might be causing this abnormality. This form of blood test specifically quantifies the response of your blood to a specific food. The ALCAT Test is itself the diagnosis and prescription for treatment—the best of all worlds.

In other words, if you test strongly positive to a food, your treatment is to avoid that food. Cut and dried: simple test, simple treatment. In our day of incredibly complicated tests and interpretations, having a blood test that tells all is a relief.

To oversimplify the value of this straightforward test would be difficult. Sometimes this raw truth can intimidate patients, who are accustomed to a medical system that often hedges rather than commit to a diagnosis and treatment. Patients are often shocked to find they are reactive to their favorite foods and the recommended treatment is to simply stop eating them. Patients hesitatingly respond, "So if I cut back on eating corn, should I lose weight?"

"No," is the answer. "If you completely eliminate all corn and corn products, you can expect all the symptoms relating to eating corn to subside."

After the initial shock has worn off, most are ready to make a rational plan to begin eliminating foods. Depending on the number of reactive foods involved, many patients can begin by eliminating a few of the most frequently eaten foods. After a week or two they should add a few more foods to their elimination list until all are included. However, they must eliminate all reactive foods to confirm whether food intolerance is or is not causing a symptom. Losing weight by spending money on eating the right food is certainly better than spending money on medication.

Feed Me

Food sensitivities may result not only in overeating, but also in malnutrition by interfering with the metabolism of fat for energy. This results in individuals who are overweight, plagued with "serotonin-boosting" cravings, and malnourished due to poor intestinal absorption of nutrients.

Exercise for these patients becomes frustrating when they consume little fat for energy and become more hungry from their exercise. When fat is not accessible to burn for energy, the body falls back on its emergency supply: the small glycogen store in the liver and muscle. Once this readily available source is used up, the body will send you to eat as quickly as possible.

If the biochemical reaction precipitated by food sensitivity blocks your metabolism of fat for energy, you repeatedly tap your emergency carbohydrate supply. Your body then insists you eat to replace this supply, and odds are slim that you will choose pure and natural carbohydrates. You are more likely to consume easily available processed food loaded with sugar and/or fat. At this point, your body is saying: "Feed me. Eat anything, and I will sort it out once it gets here." The result of this hypothetical scenario is that you will have consumed more sugar and fat that will be stored as fat, probably in the form of one or more of your favorite or reactive foods.

This perpetual cycle of living off your emergency supply of carbohydrate results in a slow but steady buildup of fat storage and the feeling of total dependence on carbohydrates for energy. Eventually your brain figures: "The only way out of this cycle is to stop exercising." So let's stop a minute and look at you.

- You have gained weight.
- When you exercise, you don't lose weight but do get hungry.
- You eat right but don't lose weight.
- You stop exercising out of frustration.
- You give in to certain foods that make you feel better.
- You have a food sensitivity!

Fat—How Did This Happen?

Like putting a figurative fence around our fat, the gate only goes into the fat cell; nothing leaves. We must eat, and inevitably, we will eat fat and sugar even as we try to eat healthily. The fat and sugar go to the fat cell through the gate guarded by the chemical response to reactive foods, never to leave again. We can store more fat, but using that fat for energy is prohibited. Imagine being allowed to buy anything you want, but once you take it into your house you can never bring it out again. With time, your only option would be to add to the size of your house. Now your friends bring you things because you have such a large house. Imagine the frustration of people continuing to bring gifts to maintain your large house when what you want is help taking the furniture and trash out.

Let's Do Lunch

Overeating as the result of an overwhelming physiologic response to an allergic chemical reaction occurring somewhere in the body is one thing. Overeating as an inappropriate immediate gratification to emotions such as stress, anger, or loneliness is another. Actually, when you consider the all-or-nothing laws of nature and physiology, you might realize that it would be abnormal to *not* overeat under certain sets of circumstances. So we manage to:

- Overeat in response to emotions—stress, anger, loneliness, or just out of blatant disregard.
- Repeatedly overuse our favorite foods on a frequent "daily" basis, which predisposes us to becoming sensitive to these foods.
- Develop chronic symptoms as a result of ongoing chemical reactions precipitated by culprit foods. (These may result from repeated overeating of foods, genetically inherited reactions to foods, or pharmacologically mediated reactions to specific chemicals in the foods.)

Somebody Do Something!

Sadly, because of lack of funds for research, we may never know the exact chemical reactions that lead us to gain and maintain weight as a response to food sensitivities. To wait idly for a satisfactory explanation for the impressive results many doctors have noticed is like refusing to tell time until we know how a watch works.

We are not talking about potentially dangerous treatments that require extensive animal and human trials for FDA approval. We are looking at a normal predictable sequence of events that can be stopped at any time by removing the figurative domino at the start of the chain reaction. After watching this reaction, preventing a repeat would seem straightforward enough—rearrange and remove some dominoes.

Domino Effect

Treating or correcting the infinite maze of reactions created by many foods we eat would seem impossible. In fact, understanding every domino, its angle and tilt, would defy the most intelligent among us. But even you and I can see that if you simply don't tip the first domino, no harm is done. The body's natural response to change is to return to a state of equilibrium. This is what saves us from evolutionarily charging blindly into a brick wall. As the body returns to "normal," the first domino now starts a spontaneous reaction that efficiently proceeds to the more beneficial outcome in the maintenance of life—without sidetracks, split pathways, and deadends, and with minimal waste of energy.

Millions of people act as they do and feel as they feel, not by choice, but because their body reacts adversely to a food they have eaten. Much like a parasitic relationship, this chemical response to normal food drains the host's reserves of energy, creates imbalances in brain chemistry, and subverts the host's energy to its purpose. To try to keep up nutritionally with this virtually continuous drain of body energy is like trying to fill a bathtub without plugging the drain.

A Gold Mine of Information

Food-sensitivity testing should be and some day will be an integral part of the thorough annual physical examination. Much of the money we currently spend on blood tests is wasted in the sense that we don't get useful information from a normal test. "Normals" for most blood tests are the cumulative averages or most common measurements in a large population sample, which is tantamount to comparing you to everybody else to decide whether you are normal. Doctors order the tests routinely and routinely discount minor abnormalities as "not important" or casually say, "we will check it again next time." If next time is a year later, how valuable was the test in the first place?

The ALCAT Test is itself the diagnosis and prescription for treatment—the best of all worlds.

In its best-case scenario, an abnormal blood test will lead to more specific tests that either confirm an otherwise undiagnosed condition or confirm that the initial test results were erroneous.

By contrast, consider routine food-sensitivity testing on an annual basis. All year long your body fights any number of conditions that cause the absorption of food through a compromised intestinal lining. These conditions may range from pregnancy to viral infection to food poisoning to yeast overgrowth to lack of digestive enzymes. The point is this: Virtually any common everyday condition can result in your body changing its reaction to a particular food.

In the ALCAT Test, the "normal" used to standard-ize the results is your own blood and cells. Thus a normal test is what's normal for you, as opposed to your being compared to a group of strangers.

Doctor, Do Something!

A food that is generally healthy for you can, a week later, set up a cascade of immune and chemical reactions in your body that have far-reaching implications if left undiagnosed. The more frequently you eat this food, the greater the strain on your systems and organs until physical symptoms may take you to your doctor. Baffled by your otherwise good health, your doctor will treat your symptoms as indicated. Unless he or she considers food sensitivities as a possible cause and does appropriate testing, your symptoms are destined to return as you continue eating the culprit food. After an appropriate number of visits, your doctor will add the adjectives "chronic" or "recurrent" in front of your original diagnosis. He or she will do further tests, change your medication, and console you in that you may require continued treatment for this problem for which there is no apparent cure.

Chronic Means "I Don't Know"

You now understand the frustrating plight of the patient with migraine headaches, sinus drainage, ear infections, overweight, irritable bowel syndrome, chronic fatigue, arthritis, and fibromyalgia, to mention a few. All these "conditions" may be merely symptoms of a body's defense system mistaking a normal food for a dangerous invader. It is to your body's credit that this protective mechanism exists and works. Unfortunately, your body uses incredible amounts of energy to protect your immune system and subsequently your organ systems when it is switched on inappropriately.

When your immune system is continuously stressed, protecting you from this food that keeps reappearing, it can no longer maintain its defenses against true invader viruses and bacteria. Likewise, nutrients otherwise destined to support other organ systems are conscripted by the immune system to support its functions. This sets in motion another cascade of events that may eventually result in symptoms of "malnutrition" or deficiencies in nutrients. As each organ system is taxed by the immune system, it may present symptoms that complicate health.

Millions of people act as they do and feel as they feel, not by choice, but because their body reacts adversely to a food they have eaten.

Unless a doctor is insightful enough to consider food sensitivities as the root cause of all your symptoms, your array of diagnoses can be numerous. Each may require medical visits and medication to control symptoms, which in turn leads to low self-esteem. As depression and frustration take over your daily life, you may well become a willing subject of the medical system that seems your only hope.

The nightmare must end. None of this had to happen. Neither you nor your kids had to miss those days of work or school. You didn't have to decline invitations or let your life revolve around medication schedules if food sensitivities were the problem. Had a relatively painless blood sample been drawn during your annual physical, you would know if you had developed sensitivities to certain foods. Long before the cascade of pathology took place, you could have prevented its progression.

Not only can you treat this problem, but treatment is less expensive than treating a chronic medical condition. Rather than buying medication and keeping doctor appointments for the rest of your life, you simply stop eating your reactive food or foods for a period of time. Often after three to six months, you can begin reintroducing these foods into your diet if you wish. All in all, you save instead of spend money to cure this condition. You stop buying your reactive foods, you add new foods to your diet, and you learn the most basic of lessons: Your health is *your* responsibility. No one knows your body better than you do. Unless you actively lead those caring for your health, you follow them.

This brings us back to my original contention, that food sensitivity testing would be more valuable than most screening tests done today. Even a negative or "normal" test reinforces your eating habits and skills and allows you to safely assume that any symptoms you develop are not food-related. Once we realize the tremendous potential food has to enrich as well as to unravel our lives, we stop taking it for granted.

The Politics of Food Sensitivities

As Scott Peck, M.D., so simply yet eloquently states in the first chapter of his book *The Road Less Traveled:* "Life is difficult." He goes on to discuss that once it is accepted that life is difficult, "the fact that life is difficult no longer matters . . . What makes life difficult is that the process of confronting and solving problems is a painful one, yet it is in this whole process of meeting and solving problems, that life has meaning." Dr. Peck puts life and the choices we make in perspective.

Those who only accept life as purely scientifically justified have long relegated the treatment of overweight to the shadows of medicine. These same individuals can offer no scientifically justified and confirmed treatment for overweight. In lieu of this, they willingly continue to treat patients' symptoms with stopgap medications. These patients are then criticized for trying to control overweight through alternative methods by the same people who offer no reliable medical treatment for their disease—an apparent "catch-22" situation. The art and the business of medicine seem to be in great conflict with regard to treating overweight. "Life *is* difficult."

Food sensitivities/allergies have been a confirmed cause of human illness since the beginning of this century when Hamburger and Schloss confirmed the first-known cases of food allergies. In that time frame, conventional medicine has accepted, denied, partially accepted, and totally denigrated food sensitivities as a true condition. This seemingly confused approach to food allergies stems from a number of issues:

- **Political**—To accept food as a cause of illness would contradict many influential scientists and divert funds from their research into curing disease with medication.

- **Medical philosophy**—Current medical doctrine is based on non-food causes of disease. For example, the symptoms of a child's cold can be traced to the release of chemicals by the immune system resulting in the release of protective body reactions to isolate and eliminate the offending agent. It is obvious that an organism is the cause of a cold because of the way our immune system reacts (or it's too difficult to consider other causes). In the era of HMOs and big business medicine, the common accepted treatment is the one that will be paid for. There is little incentive for an individual practitioner to consider patients as individuals whose common symptoms may be unrelated to the conventional "odds."

- **The wide array of symptoms caused by food allergies**—The varying symptoms related to food sensitivity perplexes the practitioner who is under pressure to give relief *now*. Americans are not given to dealing with problems for the long term; we are addicted to instant gratification. Our medical system struggles to live up to our expectations and still remain highly profitable. This precludes recommending an elimination diet that excludes what are likely your favorite foods. Since the best-case scenario—that your condition resolves and you don't need to see your doctor again—is hardly a practice-building activity, your caregiver will more likely supply the conventional medication and recommend you return if the condition doesn't improve.

- **The lack of concrete evidence as to the exact mechanisms by which food allergies perpetuate their symptoms**—This is the clincher for many physicians who need the full faith and confidence of their medical textbooks and literature behind each treatment. In all fairness, our medical/legal atmosphere perpetuates the "conventional" practice. Few physicians continue to learn with each patient they treat. Learning comes via the drug and medical equipment companies that sponsor continuing education or visit offices to update doctors on newer drugs. Drug companies seldom encourage doctors to consider something as mundane as food as the cause of and cure for patients' health problems. If you cure your migraine with food elimination, who will buy the headache medicine? If

your irritable bowel settles when you stop eating a
food, who will finance the X-ray department at the
hospital?

So as you can see, the medical establishment has little incentive to promote research into food allergies.
Even if research identified the cause of food allergies,
you can be sure that, unless big drug companies make a
pill to alleviate your symptoms, it will not be highly
touted.

Without having a complete understanding of how a
clock works, one can predictably and reliably know the
time of day. Likewise, treating food allergies is a science
of noticing the symptoms, then not noticing them once
foods are eliminated. In efforts to help patients, doctors
don't have to agree with all the intricate details of how
food allergies cause illness, but need only to be aware
that food allergies may explain their symptoms.

Do No Harm

There is no question that caution is a virtue in conventional medicine. When doctors treat a patient with a prescription medication, they must concede they usually
don't know how the medication works at the cellular level.
Therefore, they depend on careful and thorough testing
by the drug company before using the medication for patients. But this slow, time-consuming evaluation seems
overkill when applied to a therapeutic mechanism that removes a food from the diet. Asking patients to eliminate
some foods to see whether they get relief is hard enough
for doctors, but realizing that patients can cure themselves without the prescription pad is humbling.

Even those who are closed-minded regarding food-
sensitivity testing realize that some foods are more al-
lergy-provoking than others. This awareness may enable

these doctors to successfully treat many patients with food intolerance without drugs, or to relegate patient care to nutritionists, osteopaths, homeopaths, and dietitians familiar with advances in food sensitivity testing for food allergies.

Doctors for the most part do have intense concern for their patients. Sooner or later their compassion will lead them to consider the growing body of evidence that our food may be making us sick. The long-term health benefits of proper eating are undeniable, and to eat properly you must know the foods to which your body will react abnormally. Avoiding these allergic reactions is imperative to maintaining your good health.

CHAPTER 9

The Right Diet for the Twenty-first Century

For years, various doctors and other health-care professionals have noticed that patients who removed allergenic foods from their diets for any reason experienced a welcome side effect: They lost weight. Now, two breakthrough research studies have shown that this side effect is not just coincidental—they conclusively establish that eating allergenic foods contributes to weight gain in a large percentage of the population. How this occurs is not exactly understood, but research and practical experience suggest that three mechanisms are involved: the brain chemicals that trigger food addiction, the body's individual rate of metabolism, and the damage to blood vessels that causes edema.

A main reason traditional weight-loss diets often do not work is that they do not eliminate foods to which an overweight person is intolerant. The allergenic food then triggers one or more reactions, which locks the overweight person in a merciless cycle of weight gain. Any foods (and often the very foods that are craved most) can cause these problems.

Good News for Food Addicts

The good news is that when overweight people remove intolerant foods from their diet, their brain chemicals, metabolism, and digestive system normalize. Their food addictions vanish, their metabolism functions at its optimum rate, and their water retention disappears—all without the deprivation of low-calorie diets, without dangerous diet drugs, and without endless hours of exercise. What's more, groundbreaking studies on food intolerance and weight loss conducted using the ALCAT Test show that when people cut their intolerant foods from their diets, they lose not just weight, but fat, and in many cases gain lean muscle.

Kaats Research

Controlling body fat is as simple as controlling food allergies. That was the conclusion of groundbreaking research conducted in 1995 by Gilbert Kaats, Ph.D., director of the Health and Medical Research Foundation in San Antonio, Texas.

Thirty patients on a low-caloric diet plateaued. They continued low-caloric diets but also eliminated ALCAT–positive foods. Weight loss resumed and "before-and-after" body composition determinations showed that their weight loss was fat. Most interestingly, women lost fat from the hips. What you eat is more important than how much you eat. This concept upends the commonly held belief that food *quantity* is the culprit in overweight, a belief that is clearly not correct.

Addictive Overeating and Food Intolerance

The findings of these two important studies correlate with many other current studies on the relationship among individual biochemistry, food addiction, and body weight and health. Changing attitudes and new research on obesity is leading to increased interest in just what triggers overeating behavior and drives people to eat their way into obesity.

For years, psychiatrists and psychologists have observed food-addiction patterns where patients have a constant craving for food (especially candy, ice cream, and other sweets) that compels them to eat far beyond their energy requirements. They crave food like an alcoholic craves a drink or a smoker a cigarette. Doctors and weight-loss specialists have been frustrated in their efforts to help these people lose weight. Many practitioners now believe that these irresistible cravings may stem from a biochemical dependency that can sabotage any weight-control program. Allergenic foods may drive you to overeat instead of break out in a rash.

It has been suggested that obesity is associated with a defect in the appetite control system. Science is now showing us conclusively that certain foods and food chemicals trigger changes in brain chemistry that result in allergic-like addictive overeating. Dr. F. Fuller Royal, a clinical ecologist and modern day pioneer in the field of food sensitivities and environmental medicine, wrote: "I have come to realize that a very high percentage (80%) of obese patients have serious food allergy-addiction. They will never be able to adequately conquer the problems of obesity . . . until their allergic-addictive foods have been identified and eliminated from their diets." The only problem with this solution, until recently, has been identifying the offending foods. Before the ALCAT

Test, this was a difficult, expensive, and time-consuming process.

Doctors' Experiences

Doctors who use the simple ALCAT blood test have conquered the difficulties in identifying food sensitivities and are reporting such unprecedented results in helping patients control weight as the following:

> As soon as I started avoiding the foods I tested sensitive to, I began losing one to one-and-a-half pounds a week without changing my activity level or consciously reducing portions. I found I wasn't as hungry and had less cravings, so it was the easiest and most successful diet I've ever been on.
>
> —John Magauran, General Practitioner, Honolulu, Hawaii

> I tell my patients it makes sense to know your food hypersensitivities. Some of my greatest successes are members of the Austrian Ski Team, who went on to win Olympic medals.
>
> —Dr. Stephen Schimpf, Preventive Medicine and Immunotherapy, Salzburg, Austria

> We tested people who had stopped losing weight. Once we eliminated their sensitive foods they lost fat and kept it off.
>
> —Dr. Richard Bahr, Environmental Medicine, Cincinnati, Ohio

> Patients who attempt to lose weight and keep it off aren't successful until they eliminate their allergenic foods.
>
> —Dr. Barbara Solomon, Internal Medicine, Baltimore, Maryland

> One of the positive side effects of the ALCAT program for many of my patients is that they also lose weight.
>
> —Dr. Stephen Smith, Allergy and Skin, Richland, Washington

> Until I started using the ALCAT Test, I was missing some foods, chemicals, and preservatives with my patients. Now I

use it as the main instrument for testing for food allergies in a variety of conditions including weight loss, and when I can't diagnose anything definite.

—Dr. Paul Jaconello, Nutrition and
Preventive Medicine, Toronto, Ontario

We have found the ALCAT Testing and the elimination diet to be a useful tool as a part of a program to lose weight and maintain weight loss.

—James F. Bain, M.D., Family Practice,
Director of Wabash Physician Services

In my judgment, the ALCAT Test has been very useful in diagnosing food sensitivities. One of the most interesting cases is that of a young girl with eosinophilic gastroenteritis. Management of this patient was difficult until use of the ALCAT Test identified her problem foods. I have also observed that a great many of my food-sensitive patients lose weight as a result of following the exclusionary diet prescribed by the test and that this is due to something other than restriction of calorie intake.

—Leland Green, M.D., Board Certified Allergist,
Lansdale, Pennsylvania

I have never found anything better for diagnosing food sensitivities in children than the ALCAT Test. I have used it extensively for many years and have found it to be especially helpful with the more complicated cases. It is also very useful for identifying adverse reactions to the food additives, chemicals, and antibiotics. The potential effects of these substances is a very important consideration.

—Walter Ward, M.D., ENT Allergy and Environmental Medicine,
Winston-Salem, North Carolina

Beyond the Zone

One interesting note comes from Barry Sears through his popular book *The Zone,* in which he discusses the important relationship of hormones to obesity. His complex theory revolves around certain superhormones called eicosanoids. Actually, eicosanoids are not technically hormones but autacoids, since they exert their effect locally in the tissue in which they are formed rather than systemically as circulating hormones. This particular aspect of eicosanoids makes their application to food intolerance that much more practical. One perplexing aspect of food intolerance has been its seemingly inconsistent presentation of symptoms in a variety of organ systems. This is now clarified by understanding that tissues have different eicosanoid binding sites. That is, certain eicosanoids affect certain tissues preferentially. Depending on the particular eicosanoid reaction to food intolerance, symptoms may appear as gastrointestinal, respiratory, vascular, or dermatological. For that matter, any organ system may be affected.

Certain eicosanoids are produced in adipose tissue and are potent regulators of the breakdown of fat. In particular PGE-2 (prostaglandin E-2) inhibits lipolysis. That means it prevents the breakdown of fat for energy. Anything that increases the synthesis of this eicosanoid may prevent you from using your own fat stores for energy, regardless of how much you exercise. Add to this the anti-lipolytic (also inhibits lipolysis) effect of insulin, and you may become a carbohydrate junkie to meet your basic metabolic energy requirements. Also synthesized by adipose tissue is PGI-2. This eicosanoid promotes the breakdown of fat and is lipolytic in its action. The coordinated modulation of these two eicosanoids results in what most of us consider normal fat metabolism. But when one eicosanoid is synthesized preferentially over the other, an imbalance of fat metabolism occurs.

Who Are Those Guys?

Eicosanoids are arachidonic acid metabolites. Arachidonic acid is an essential fatty acid that must be supplied in the diet, as the body has no way of deriving it from normal metabolic pathways. Arachidonic acid exists in the plasma membrane of all cells. Eicosanoid synthesis would seem to be dependent on a variety of chemically and hormonally mediated events. The particular eicosanoids synthesized in a tissue are determined by the enzyme systems present in that tissue. Thus, some eicosanoids may affect many cells, albeit in different ways. Others may exert their effect in only a few select tissues.

What Does This Have to Do with Food?

Food intolerance results in an inflammatory reaction mediated by the immune system. Inflammation results in or from the synthesis of eicosanoids. For example, the polymorphonuclear white blood cells that engulf and destroy allergenic food particles release PGE-2. Furthermore, PGE-2 depresses lymphocyte function and may result in depressed cellular immunity. PGE-2 also causes vasodilatation and increased vascular permeability. This results in local tissue edema and fluid retention. PGE-2 has known adverse effects on fat metabolism, blood vessel permeability, insulin production, gastric acid output, platelet aggregation, and bronchoconstriction and can result in immune system suppression, dysmenorrhea, and inflammation. If all this can come from a reaction to a food, we are far beyond worrying whether eating ice cream would ruin our diet.

Why Hasn't Anyone Told Me?

Throughout this book we have stressed the need for further research into the relationship of food intolerance and chronic disease. Before such research is concluded, thousands of eicosanoids may be identified. The example of PGE-2 used here may be only a start. Even today many eicosanoids are recognized whose function and activity are uncertain. The question is: Do you want to learn how to make a watch or do you want to know what time it is?

The point is that for now it is only interesting to know the postulated mechanism by which food intolerance may affect overweight and other chronic conditions. Forget about how it happens; just realize it *is* happening. Realize that you control the reactions that take place in your body by the foods you choose to eat.

How Does It Work?

What we take for granted as a "normal" diet is a relatively recent cultural development. For one thing, until recently people in many parts of the world were never exposed to foods not indigenous to their area. In some instances, the modern diet has outstripped biological mechanisms of adaptation. As was previously mentioned, members of certain ethnic groups have not evolved the digestive enzymes needed to fully digest cow's milk protein, a relatively recent evolutionary event. According to Harrison's *Principles of Internal Medicine*, "It would appear that about 5 to 15 percent of the adult white population shows intestinal lactase deficiency, but in black Americans, Bantus, and Orientals, the incidence has been reported as high as 80 to 90 percent."

In the last 50 years our diet has changed dramatically. The same digestive enzymes that were needed to digest only fresh fruits and vegetables and range-fed meats must now somehow deal with the huge amounts of preservatives, colorings, chemical fertilizers, insecticides, and antibiotics in our foods. As our digestive enzymes fall short, our immune systems react to these substances to protect us from the toxic consequences.

Food intolerance knocks the body's biochemistry out of balance. As a result, the metabolism becomes sluggish, the immune system becomes impaired, the digestive tract develops leaks, insulin and other hormones become imbalanced, and the body loses control of the neurotransmitters that control appetite. Your brain assimilates all this and sends the message: "You are falling apart."

There are no universally safe foods, with the possible exception of pure water.

When the chemicals that control appetite are altered, they trigger food cravings and eating binges; when normal metabolism is disrupted, it impacts how much fat is stored; and when the vascular system is damaged, it causes fluid to leak into connective tissues, which results in water retention. All in all, not a pretty picture. But there's hope. Research studies using the ALCAT Test have shown that once you take care of your food intolerances, the body is able to lose fat. It's suspected that by removing the food disruptions, the body's mechanisms normalize, resulting in a reduction in the body's physiological craving for sweets and carbohydrates, normalization of the body's hunger mechanisms, and a return to efficient fat burning. What's more, with these food disturbances out of your system, you will feel healthier and more energetic. This increases the chance that you will exercise.

No One Size Fits All Diet

Overweight people share one common denominator—they have too much stored fat tissue. Their paths to overweight may be as randomly different as snowflakes. And yet many cookie-cutter diets are touted. Who's looking out for the individual? Few recognize the powerful mechanisms that make each person unique—for example, inherited difference of hormones and metabolism; environmental variations in exposure to pollution; lifestyle differences of stress; and particular food choices impacting the individual. The key is to understand and adapt the diet to the powerful forces that help to determine body weight.

Following a weight-loss diet that instructs you to eat one orange, an egg, and toast for breakfast may sound healthy and well balanced. But what if you're intolerant to eggs? What if that very egg you ate caused your blood cells to expand and explode, and this reaction caused your serotonin level to plummet and send a message from your brain to eat more carbohydrate? You're going to find it hard to lose weight on that diet. The problem seems to arise from the fact that some foods have been declared universally healthy by popular acclaim. There are no universally safe foods, with the possible exception of pure water.

Because you are not a clone of your neighbor, you need a diet that takes your uniqueness into consideration.

If you're intolerant to tuna, you don't have tuna sandwiches for lunch no matter what your friend eats. Clothes look different on your body, perfumes smell different on your skin, and food acts different inside. *Vive la différence!*

If we truly intend to treat obesity as the medical problem it is claimed to be, how can one dietary solution work for every person? Other medical problems do not have a single solution. When treating other diseases and conditions, doctors take into account each patient's medical history, degree of illness, reaction to pharmaceuticals, and other information. Then they design a treatment plan for that person. Weight loss deserves the same one-on-one attention since no two people are genetically, biochemically, or psychologically the same.

Obesity is recognized as a chronic medical condition because of its impact on other organ systems and overall health. Its solution, however, may lie in the use of less medication. The identification of reactive foods and their avoidance may represent the indicated medical treatment for this "plague." So many subtle functions within the cells defend the body from the effects of the minute but powerful eicosanoids. These trigger waves of hormonal activity, and the expulsion of powerful mediating chemicals, which go about the task of eliminating or neutralizing invaders, like law enforcement officers with stun guns at a riot.

Now we have a scientifically proven method for identifying offending foods and food substances that can be applied to a broad range of programs and have a profound effect in reducing health-care costs.

Drugs are for the most part very effective clinically, but they work from outside the body's basic chemistry to affect only hunger or cravings. They have a number of drawbacks in terms of side effects, cost, and the need for long-term use to artificially modulate hunger and cravings. They fail to keep weight off long-term if food intolerances are not identified and eliminated.

Candida yeast infection has also been shown to be a factor in weight gain. In particular, because it causes the body to crave sugar, which feeds the candida yeast, causing them to grow. It also increases production of insulin, which pushes the sugar out of the bloodstream and deposits it, as fat, into the fat cells. Intestinal yeast infections are a known risk factor in the development of food intolerance. Treating the yeast without considering the possibility of food intolerance is only partially treating a person's overweight problem.

Recognize its importance to you and drink water instead of the chemical liquid convenience drinks.

Low-calorie diets work initially but weight regain is all too often speedier than the weight loss was, if a person has unidentified food intolerances.

Intense aerobic exercise should control excess fat but often fails to meet expectations if a person has unidentified food intolerance. Exercise alone has rarely been successful in eliminating excess body fat. It must be accompanied by dietary adjustments, and it is impossible to know which foods to eat until you know your food intolerances.

So, you see, while other aspects of controlling and maintaining weight may all have a place, knowing your food limitations is the secret to controlling your overweight. Everyone needs to exercise in some fashion, even if that just means moving around more. Diet drugs may be useful in defraying the urges to overeat while you focus on eliminating foods that cause cravings. Reasonable calorie control is obviously necessary to prevent weight gain. And control of candidiasis is useful in alleviating some sweet cravings and correcting intestinal function. But food intolerance and the subtle effects it has on eicosanoids, insulin, the thyroid, serotonin, the immune system, nutrient absorption, and digestion are a whole different dimension from overeating food because it looks or tastes good.

What makes any program work better, what holds it all together, is knowing and understanding your food intolerances.

One Simple Blood Test

Unfortunately, we may never know the exact chemical reactions that lead to weight gain and maintenance of overweight as a result of food intolerance because we lack funds for research. But to wait idly for a satisfactory explanation for the impressive results would deny millions the potential for improving their lives.

The ALCAT Test has a great track record. Many studies and reports substantiate it as the premier test to determine foods to which the individual is intolerant. A state-of-the-art evolution of blood tests that evaluate the individual's cellular response to an allergic substance, the test consists of making measurements of white blood cells and platelets in an individual's blood specimen. The whole blood is then exposed to common food extracts and chemicals. The specific reaction of the cells to these foods and chemicals then tells the story. Changes occur in these blood cells if they have been programmed by the body to react to the food and chemicals in question. By detecting and quantifying the degree of change in the blood cells, the ALCAT Test then determines the degree of reactivity the tested individual has to the substance.

Because each determination is calibrated to the individual's own blood, there is no "normal" to look up in a book. In other words, a normal response is the response of the same individual's blood before the food or chemical is introduced. The ALCAT Test's highly individualized nature makes it preferable over tests that report results in the broad "normal" range for the general population. Confirmation comes through the relief of symptoms as one eliminates the culprit foods from the diet. The simplicity of the concept belies how intricate the actual process is. This is pure medicine, in that curing the disease rather than covering it up relieves symptoms.

We are not talking potentially dangerous treatments or drugs that require extensive trials and studies to confirm their safety. We are talking common sense that confounds the tenets of scientific investigation. After all, what is common sense to one is heresy to another. But while the purists study, and while the drug companies seek further ways to profit, you and I can heal ourselves by understanding that food may be causing many of our miseries and by avoiding the foods that do.

Piecing the Puzzle Together

As we cruise into the twenty-first century, we have to reverse the terrible trends associated with obesity. This can be done in the conventional way by treating each symptom as it appears or it can be done the ALCAT way—accepting food intolerance as a real disease and treating the cause to reduce the incidence of symptoms: obesity, ADD, migraines, irritable bowel syndrome, colitis, depression, reflux gastritis, arthritis, and sinusitis, among others. During most of the twentieth century, these were considered diseases that had no real cure and could only be treated symptomatically. Medicine now knows that in many cases they were only symptoms of the underlying condition of food intolerance.

The next century will find us using selective food elimination and consumption to improve the quality of our lives. Simple blood tests like the ALCAT Test will guide us through the maze of available foods.

But don't wait! Start now to use food as your medicine. If you are now trying to lose weight or contemplating starting a weight-loss program, learn your food intolerances. Super-charge any sensible weight-loss program and make it last by understanding food intolerance and its cure. Lose weight by applying yourself diligently to limiting unnecessary calories, taking in plenty of nutrient, and avoiding your reactive foods. Finally, a practical solution: Avoid your reactive foods, and cravings will disappear, leaving you to concentrate on eating foods that will supply nutrient. Energy levels will improve and exercise will become a realistic option. Think clearly, run faster, and love living.

The new hunter-gatherer searches in earnest for nutrient to maximize his or her potential and shuns food that limits his or her mental and physical well-being. "Thou shalt not eat of the forbidden fruit." And the forbidden fruit is determined by your body's reaction to foods you choose. Know your forbidden foods and avoid them.

Nutrient-Driven Eating

One outstanding feature of the ALCAT Test is that, along with identifying your reactive foods, it reports your safe foods as well. This means you not only have a good idea which foods may be making you sick, but also have a ready selection to use in lieu of your reactive foods. This is especially important for cases in which the food to be eliminated represents a substantial source of a particular vitamin or mineral. For example, if carrots were found reactive and were your only significant source of beta-carotene, eliminating them could result in a serious deficiency of vitamin A in your body.

On the other hand, with guidance, you will be able to identify several other rich sources of beta-carotene among the list of "safe" foods in the ALCAT report manual. Minerals likewise must be accounted for if rich sources are eliminated. For example, if you eliminate milk, taking calcium supplements or choosing to eat calcium-rich "safe" foods would be wise.

Although most of us feel uncomfortable with the responsibility of replacing deficient vitamins and minerals in our bodies, we shouldn't. That is what eating is. The fact that we willingly delegate our nutritional replenishment to the short-order cook at the fast-food restaurant is the epitome of irresponsibility. To regain control of our health, we must reclaim responsibility for what we eat. Hidden food allergies begin all too often as a result of mindless eating of nutrient-depleted processed foods on a daily basis. We often eat only our favorite foods, eat too fast, and eat for reasons other than hunger.

Rotate, Rotate, Rotate

Blind luck would give us better nutrition if we varied our food choices from day to day. The rotation diet concept has long been a standard for avoiding the development of food intolerance. As a general rule, avoid eating a food more often than every fourth day, and your chances of developing food intolerance diminish. In our fast-food–dependent society, this takes more planning than just eating at a different restaurant each day. We must give especially careful thought to avoiding foods such as wheat, corn, milk, soy, and eggs because they appear in so many different forms of fast food. As a matter of fact, eating out becomes a greater hassle than it is worth as we attempt to avoid foods we know are bad for us. As an aid, the ALCAT Test results include a four-day planned rotation diet from the theoretically "safe foods."

But I Take a Multivitamin

A healthy body is the result of careful planning. On our behalf, the Food and Drug Administration has calculated the amounts of various vitamins and minerals necessary to prevent deficiency states. The recommended amounts necessary to keep from showing signs of deficiency are reported as RDA, or Recommended Daily Allowances, as standards for food labeling. To me, the thought of taking just enough vitamin C to keep scurvy away seems a bit passive.

Recently, the *University Wellness Letter,* a well-known health reference, has recommended vitamin C doses of 500 mg per day and vitamin E of 400 to 800 mg per day. This represents a shift away from minimum doses to prevent signs of deficiency and a groundswell toward doses of vitamins and nutrients to therapeutically promote health. More important, this suggests some useful research may be forthcoming regarding using nutrients to prevent disease.

First of all, the human body gets its most usable form of nutrients, vitamins, and minerals from fruits, seeds, nuts, vegetables, unprocessed grains, meat, and fish. Other sources are less usable by the body. Artificial supplements should not be taken in lieu of eating properly but to enhance the body's ability to fight disease. Taking vitamins to substitute for eating carefully is like substituting a Ford Pinto for a limousine. It may get you there, but it just won't be the same, and you won't feel nearly as good.

So don't choke down the one-a-day vitamin and think you have done your duty. Your intestine likely will treat it like the candy-armored nugget it is and may chip the porcelain off the toilet bowl. Take your vitamin and mineral supplements at various times during the day and be sure they are likely to dissolve in your gut. (Your pills should dissolve in 30 minutes in vinegar if they are likely to do you any good at all!) Our intestine is designed to absorb a steady stream of nutrients all day, so present your supplements in this way.

Feeding the Immune System

As one recovers from the often devastating effects of food intolerance, recognizing and correcting deficiencies that have developed in the body is also important. Eliminating the culprit foods gives the immune system some respite, some breathing room, if you will. The problem is that the damage has been done to some extent.

The various immune cells have been overworked for some period of time. This has set in place the natural cascade of reactions that follows depletion of immune cell nutrients. This sequence of reactions can result in misfiring of the immune system cells. Since the network of cells making up your immune system depends on continuous communication, failure of any part of your system may result in a rogue immune system that may attack your body itself. This autoimmune destruction of body tissues is classic in many chronic diseases. Rather than selectively treating these autoimmune diseases, you would do well to initiate nutritional resuscitation of the immune system so as to minimize permanent damage to your body tissues.

Even before your food intolerance is completely resolved, it is important that you begin rehabilitating your weakened immune system. Assuming poor absorption from the intestinal tract, supplementing vitamins and minerals vital to assure healthy immune system functioning is warranted. These supplements, combined with an appropriate elimination diet, will begin to normalize the digestion, absorption, and metabolism of nutrients needed to correct conditions brought about by immune system attacks on the body itself. Keep in mind that the malnourished and overactive immune system leads to many symptoms of food intolerance.

Some well-established immune system nutrients and suggested supplemental dosages are as follows:

Vitamin E   400mg/day is generally accepted as safe. This powerful antioxidant is a confirmed immune-system potentiator. It is important to use only D-alpha tocopherol and avoid DL-alpha tocopherol, which the body is not able to assimilate well (Think of "DL" as "Don't Like").

Vitamin C   1000mg/day in divided doses is conservative and up to 10,000mg/day may be justified in times of illness as the body consumes enormous amounts under stress. Every immune system function benefits from the presence of vitamin C. Diarrhea is an upper limit sign and the dose should be decreased until diarrhea resolves.

Beta Carotene 15mg/day or 25,000 units/day are recommended. This precursor to vitamin A is a highly regarded immune system stimulant. Several studies have documented its benefits in protecting from cancer, and it is necessary for some immune cells to mature properly.

Selenium 100–200mg/day. This potent antioxidant teams up with vitamin E to protect cells.

B vitamins This group of vitamins is best taken in a "complex" containing the range of B vitamins. Vitamin B6 is especially susceptible to deficiency from poor absorption. University studies confirm that vitamin B6 plays an important role in the immune system.

Zinc 50mg/day of this mineral is invaluable for immune cell development and activity. Immune system activity consumes large quantities of zinc. Zinc supplements should be taken separate from multivitamin supplements since copper and iron may inhibit the absorption of zinc.

Calcium 1000mg/day. This mineral is necessary for the activation of complement, a component of the immune system which works with antibodies to destroy bacteria.

Magnesium 500mg/day is recommended. Deficiency depresses immunoglobulins needed to fight bacterial and viral infection.

Copper 3 mg/day. The exact role of copper is not known but deficiency leads to suppressed immune function.

Iron Dosage should be individualized based on documented deficiency by laboratory tests. Deficiency leads to decreased T cells.

These dosages are guidelines only and individual requirements will vary. All vitamin and mineral supplements should be labeled "corn, milk, wheat, soy, sugar, and yeast free." Your doctor or health-care professional may have further recommendations depending on your particular needs.

Each of these nutrients is found in a healthy diet of meat, fruits, and vegetables. But under the circumstances of potential intestinal malabsorption, supplemental doses are indicated to improve their availability. Also, in some cases elimination diets result in unintended deficiencies of some nutrients that must be supplemented until the food is reintroduced. It is important that you understand that long-standing food intolerance may result in a number of physiologic disturbances, which must be corrected before you will feel your best. This will take time, but now that you are eating healthy, you have all the time in the world.

For those interested in taking a more active part in their nutritional well-being, the *Encyclopedia of Nutritional Supplements,* by Michael T. Murray, N.D., is an excellent reference. Developmental studies adapting the ALCAT Test to determine individual nutritional needs are currently underway. This will permit individualized evaluation of nutrient deficiencies from a blood specimen.

The immune system has been shown to benefit from a variety of activities—music, regular physical exercise, deep breathing exercises, laughter, a positive mental attitude, and regular sleep patterns. Take a minute and look at this list of great ideas that are healthy to boot, and think of ways you can further incorporate them into your life.

Several herbal remedies and tonics may be beneficial to the immune system. Although laboratory information regarding the exact effects of herbs on the immune system is scarce, enough of us have recognized their healing powers to warrant their inclusion here. Among the common herbs and natural supplements that have a beneficial impact on the immune system are:

- Garlic
- Ginseng
- Echinacea
- Astragalus
- Spirulina (actually a food)

Because doses of these products are variable, you may find it helpful to discuss their use with a practitioner who is acquainted with their benefits in order to achieve the best results. The human body contains as many mysteries as there are foods. We'll figure them out later; just get well now. Once you correct nutrient deficiencies and food sensitivities, you are equipped to experience life to the fullest. You may be surprised at how good you feel every day now.

Eating to Avoid Food Intolerance: Rotate It

Once food sensitivities have occupied a place in your life, you will be eager to avoid them in the future. Although there is no fail-safe method to prevent the development of new food sensitivities, some practical precautions can help. Ideally, planning meals in such a way as to avoid eating the same food more often than every four days is an excellent preventive. This allows your body to recoup its immune forces between exposures, and such rare exposure to the food antigen is unlikely to perpetuate food intolerance. This technique has the added benefit of incorporating a wider variety of foods into the diet for nutrient purposes.

Save Your Enzymes

Using supplemental digestive enzymes may improve your digestion of food. As mentioned earlier, your body will not develop intolerance to the individual amino acids and fatty acids in food. Thorough digestion is without question important in preventing food intolerance. Although digestive enzyme deficiency is common in the elderly, enzyme deficiency may also occur in younger people who overeat.

Our modern diet, composed of highly processed foods, places an enormous demand on our digestive enzymes. These boxed and packaged foods are "dead food." The living, natural enzymes originally present in the food have been killed by processing. This means that the body must bear the entire enzymatic burden for digestion. Eating such food day after day creates a tremendous drain on our digestive resources. Add to this the enormous quantities of food that are commonly consumed with a chew and a swallow in our fast-paced lives, and the digestive enzymes our body has allotted for a meal are soon overwhelmed. This results in large quantities of incompletely digested food entering our intestine for absorption.

This mass of partially digested food is the cornerstone of food intolerance. Any disruption in the integrity of the absorptive surface of the intestine may allow the actual absorption of this undigested food into the bloodstream. On the other hand, if the food had been well digested, even less than ideal intestinal conditions would have allowed only well-digested food particles to be absorbed. Since the immune system selectively ignores the small components of well-digested food, immune mediated allergic reactions are avoided.

In the Raw

Eat slowly, chew food well, and eat as much raw food as possible. Raw food retains enzymes that begin assisting in digestion as soon as chewing begins. This improves the efficiency of our own enzymes since the body only secretes the amount of enzyme needed to completely digest a food. If natural enzymes are present in the food, the body will need to secrete fewer of its own precious enzymes to finish the job.

Raw food, however, contains only enough enzymes for its own digestion. The enzymes of raw food cannot be expected to contribute to the digestion of "dead" or processed food. Utilization of our enzyme stores for digestion leaves fewer enzymes available to carry out normal metabolic processes, such as tissue repair and detoxification. Once the value of digestive enzymes is appreciated, supplemental enzymes are recognized for the bargain they are. If supplemental enzymes are used, they should be of "pharmaceutical" grade and not the commercial grade found in most health-food stores. The AMTL Company, provider of the ALCAT Test, has available a high-quality enzyme supplement to benefit those who are food intolerant.

Keep Food Simple

As I have mentioned before, rotating foods is an integral part of avoiding food intolerance. To do this, you must concentrate on eating simple foods—pure, straightforward dishes. Put aside the exotic mystique of ethnic foods for the time being. These foods and even many American concoctions contain a large number of different foods in each dish. This makes varying foods on a daily basis difficult.

For example, after eating a routine Mexican food dinner, you could easily find yourself needing to avoid wheat, corn, tomatoes, milk, chicken, peppers, onions, beans, cheese, rice, eggs, avocados, and brewers yeast for a period of three days. In one fell swoop the next three days' eating is severely limited. Careful planning, however, can yield tasty and well-rounded simple meals for all four days.

Processed Food Is Dead Food

Packaged, highly processed convenience foods resemble their natural namesake only in name. Skeletonized of nutrient, these foods pose a threat to health because of their tendency to provoke intolerance. The high chemical and preservative content of processed foods qualify them to stay on the shelf—so leave them there. Common sense dictates avoiding these pseudo-foods and returning to foods in their nutritionally rich natural form.

Timing Is Everything

It takes an estimated 20 minutes for the brain to get the message from the stomach that hunger is no longer a problem. This may not sound scientific, but nonetheless it is a simplified version of the feedback mechanisms of hormones released following the absorption of macronutrient (basically fat, carbohydrate, or protein). The body is programmed to assume that when you eat you are eating naturally occurring foods. In these, the macronutrient is a carrier for various micronutrients, which are the "personality" of your body systems.

Micronutrients include vitamins, minerals, trace elements, co-enzymes, and enzymes—all found naturally in unprocessed foods. When provided the appropriate amount of micronutrient, each system operates at its peak efficiency. Deficiencies of micronutrient may result in cravings or hunger. One particularly bizarre example of this is iron deficiency; those who lack sufficient iron may crave substances such as starch, ice, and clay. The physiologic basis of this condition, known as pica, is not understood. However, the fact that a micronutrient deficiency can create an abnormal hunger is thought-provoking.

As mentioned earlier, the recognized feedback mechanisms for hunger depend on intake of macronutrient. Allowing the body the necessary time to digest and absorb macronutrient to satisfy hunger is crucial. It takes about 20 minutes for the "no-longer-hungry" or satiety signal to get from the stomach to the brain. And we all know how much damage can be done to a plate of food in 20 minutes. Macronutrient, as previously defined, is the body's source of calories. It is also the body's source of allergic reactions. I know of no research suggesting allergic reactions resulting from naturally occurring vitamins or minerals (micronutrient). At any rate, allowing at least 20 minutes for eating allows your enzymatic digestion to keep pace and stopping eating when your hunger subsides prevents overtaxing the digestive capacity. Get in the habit of leaving food on the plate.

Water, Water Everywhere, and Not Enough Is Drunk

Water is the elixir of youth. It serves more functions in the body than a secretary in a busy real-estate office. Drinking water helps fill the stomach and decrease hunger. While washing waste out of the intestine as a natural laxative, water also maintains the integrity of the cardiovascular system, speeds the removal of waste and toxins through the liver and kidneys, enhances the appearance of skin, and functions in innumerable chemical reactions in the body. Water dilutes adverse chemical reactions in the bloodstream and speeds their elimination; it also hydrates the skin and mucous membranes, including the intestinal lining. A person may live an estimated 30 days without food, but only three days without water. Recognize its importance to you and drink water instead of the chemical liquid convenience drinks.

There is much controversy regarding the safety of different water supplies. Chlorine is an excellent additive to water until it reaches your lips. As you increase your water intake, use filtered water or bottled spring water to minimize exposure to unnecessary chemicals. These sources are not unconditionally safe, but overall are a better choice, in my opinion, than chlorinated water.

The chlorine in municipal water supplies is toxic to the beneficial bacteria of the intestines. These bacteria perform important digestive functions for us in exchange for a place to live. Undue elimination of these bacteria may increase the likelihood that yeast will colonize in the intestines. These parasites may disturb absorption and predispose us to food intolerance by virtue of their effect on the intestinal lining.

Drink between two and three liters of water a day to supply the body with all it needs for a full day's work. If you have unusual conditions such as congestive heart failure or kidney disease, ask your doctor before increasing your water intake. But even with such conditions, sodas, coffee, and tea are not substitutes for pure water.

When Intolerant, Do As Intolerants Do

If you are intolerant of a food, take a proactive stance in avoiding it. It doesn't matter whether you eat a reactive food intentionally or out of ignorance; the results will be the same. Knowledge is power, but knowledge is impotent unless implemented. Once you know your reactive foods, use this greater power to control your health.

Don't Mess with Mother Intestine

The rate-limiting factor in the development of food intolerance is the intestinal lining. As long as it is intact and functioning properly, food intolerance is less likely to develop. Since food intolerance usually involves the body's immune system recognizing a food particle as foreign, absorbing only completely digested food across the intestinal lining would preclude most adverse reactions to foods, except those that are pharmacologically mediated or toxic. As mentioned previously, the immune system will not react to individual amino acids, fatty acids, or very small carbohydrate particles.

Avoid unnecessary doses of aspirin and non-steroidal anti-inflammatories, as they have a direct effect on the intestinal wall and may predispose you to food intolerance. Overindulging in alcoholic beverages is known to irritate the gastrointestinal tract. Overusing antibiotics will disrupt the natural balance of gut flora. Anything that disturbs your intestine, in fact, may predispose you to food intolerance.

CHAPTER 10

Airways and Food Intolerance

There is no feeling more terrifying than running out of oxygen. Allergic airway disease may be due to food intolerance as well as airborne allergens. Yet of conditions traditional doctors believe are *not* helped by addressing a person's food intolerance, airway problems—including asthma, hay fever, and sinusitis—top the list. The general belief is that these conditions are caused almost exclusively by inhalant allergies. But as already mentioned, nothing is simple in the world of allergy and food intolerance. By excluding a diagnosis of food intolerance from the possible causes of respiratory ailments, physicians could be allowing several million people to suffer more than is necessary each year.

Breathing Easier

But luckily for many people, some doctors do take the link between food and respiratory problems into consideration.

Gretchen, Moselle, Stacey, Christian, and Patricia, whose cases are given below, are a few people who now breathe easier because their doctors recognize the powerful impact food intolerance can have on any illness, including respiratory problems. Groundbreaking research is also showing that testing for food intolerance is a promising therapy for the millions who suffer from respiratory problems, and who long to breathe easier once again.

Enjoying Springtime for the First Time

Gretchen is among the grateful former sinus sufferers who lived for years with hay fever and asthma. She was so happy to be free of a dripping nose, stuffy sinus, and labored breathing spells that she wrote to thank Just Hintz, the director of an ALCAT Testing Laboratory in Germany, for helping her regain her health.

> I would like to thank you for what you have given me with your allergy test. You've given me symptom-free springs. In previous years, I suffered in the most beautiful time of the year with very aggressive hay fever which kept me awake for many nights and which was also the origin of my asthma. Since I was not able to breathe well on my own, an inhalator was my constant partner. Therapeutic nose drops didn't bring any relief. The worst part of my condition was not being able to breathe and the helplessness of not being able to do anything about it.
>
> I could not accept this helplessness and I started reading about allergies. Quickly, I realized that it was not only the pollen that could be causing my suffering, but food allergy could also be the origin of my symptoms. In my research, I read about your ALCAT Test, and after giving it careful thought, I decided to do the test. I can only say, thank God. Since avoiding the foods to which I'm allergic, including the most severe—grains—I have no more symptoms. I'm reminded of the benefit of the test every time I cheat on my diet. For example, if I take even a little bite of a roll at Sunday breakfast, for the next two days I'll have a dripping nose.

Like many people, Gretchen was one of the lucky hay fever and asthma suffers who learned that foods were either causing or exacerbating her respiratory problems. Unfortunately, millions of others have not yet been tested for the possibility. "Because this relationship between food and the nose is not widely recognized by most conventional doctors, few patients with this problem get satisfactory treatment," wrote Dr. Jonathan Brostoff in his book *Hayfever: The Complete Guide.* "And because the symptoms do not come on as soon as they eat the food, the patients themselves are generally unaware of the connection." He agrees that food intolerance is worth considering as a therapy for people suffering from respiratory problems, considering the growing numbers of people who are already being helped.

The Breath of Life

Moselle doesn't even want to think about where she would be today if a doctor hadn't finally diagnosed food intolerance as the cause of her recurrent sinusitis, a condition she'd suffered for five years. The chronic sinus condition had become particularly severe following a bad cold and a ruptured eardrum in 1984. Within months, her health deteriorated to the point that she had to quit her job as a registered nurse. So fatigued by her condition that she didn't have the energy to take care of her house any longer, she was also forced to move from her beloved home into a small condominium. "I couldn't keep up with the everyday activities of living," she explains. Over five years, Moselle saw three ear, nose, and throat specialists, and she was constantly on antibiotics. "As soon as the effect of one antibiotic wore off, I would get another sinus infection." At one point she was even in the hospital for ten days on intravenous penicillin. She also had to have surgery to fix a deviated septum that developed from her affliction.

Despite all these medical treatments, Moselle's health continued a downhill slide—until the day she visited Dr. Barbara Solomon and was tested for food intolerance. Moselle explains:

> It turned my whole life around. I had tried to address my sinus condition through conventional means and mainstream doctors. They experimented with all sorts of methods on me, but since none of the treatments were working I'd gotten to the point that I believed I was going to have to live for the rest of my life with breathing problems, headaches, and fatigue. I was very skeptical when I first came to Dr. Solomon and she told me that she thought she could help me, because all of the other doctors had said they could help me, too. The first thing she addressed was food allergy, which was very foreign to me. But I went on a diet that eliminated all of my food allergens, including corn, wheat, yeast, sugar, and milk, and I was better almost immediately. Within a year I started looking for a new home. With my health back, the condominium had become too boring. Now I'm able to do gardening again and do all of the things I love doing. I even took a part-time nursing job—with Dr. Solomon.

The Trouble with Asthma

Asthma, hay fever, and sinusitis are among the most common allergy complaints today. Asthma, in particular, is on the rise. This potentially dangerous disease is thought to be compounded by our increasingly polluted and chemically adulterated modern world. Twelve million people suffer from asthma in the U.S. alone. Of these, five thousand die every year. In fact, mortality has doubled since 1978, with people who live in cities being the hardest hit. The characteristic symptoms of asthma, which include wheezing, coughing, shortness of breath, and chest tightness, are produced by a constriction of the air passages.

This happens when an allergen triggers IgE anti-bodies in the mast cells of the bronchial tubes, which lead from the trachea to the lungs. The antibodies cause the mast cells to release their powerful chemicals—including the well-known chemical mediator histamine. This causes inflammation of the membranes lining the tubes. The tubes then become thicker and produce more mucus, which restricts the passage of air. A full-blown asthma attack occurs when so many chemicals are released from the mast cells that the smooth muscles of the bronchial tubes contract and become narrow, making a fresh breath of air increasingly difficult.

Today's medical treatments for asthma are surprisingly disappointing, considering asthma's prevalence and rate of growth. Therapy typically involves a series of drugs including bronchodilators and anti-inflammatories. However, among the drawbacks of these medications are their short-lived effects and serious side effects, including fogginess, fatigue, even death. Long-term use of steroids poses serious risk of adrenal suppression and other complications, including weight gain. As in many conditions the response of modern medicine to asthma leaves the sufferer contemplating this question: Is the cure worse than the disease?

Common Airway Conditions

Along with asthma, two other respiratory conditions—hay fever (also known as allergic rhinitis) and sinusitis—are common. Combined, these two respiratory conditions affect an estimated 14 million Americans. Hay fever, which is caused by pollens such as ragweed, affects as many as one in five Americans. In hay fever sufferers, pollen triggers the mast cells of the tissues that come into contact with the environment (including the nose, throat, and eyes) by releasing mediators that cause inflammation of the delicate tissues. Sufferers experience this reaction as red, itchy, watery eyes, and a runny or congested nose. Although usually seasonal, affecting a person when his particular allergen or allergens are in season, hay fever can also be exacerbated by food.

Sinusitis is an unpleasant and often painful infection of the air-filled bony cavities that surround the nasal passages. It is caused by the inflammation that occurs with hay fever and the common cold. The main symptoms of sinusitis are a severely blocked nose, headache over the eyes, or an ache in the cheeks. For some people, like Moselle, a severe case of sinusitis can completely decimate their quality of life.

Food intolerance triggers the body by different mechanisms than traditional airborne and traditional food allergy. One theory is that in a person with food intolerance the food allergen, combined with an airborne allergy, puts additional stress on the body and it collapses under the load, such as Moselle did.

Identifying the Thieves of Good Health

Of course, like Moselle, some lucky people find that by avoiding their intolerant foods, they find a cure for their airway conditions, or at the very least, reduce the impact of their problems. Like Moselle, Patricia was stunned to learn that the very foods she ate every day were ruining her health. She had suffered for years with asthma and eczema, when she finally found Dr. John W. Gerrard, an allergy and immunology specialist and former Professor of Pediatrics at the University of Saskatchewan in Canada. Although she suffered extensively from both conditions, she never associated the onset of a bout of asthma or skin rash with the particular foods she was eating. In fact, she says that if she'd had to guess which foods were aggravating her health problems, she would never have presumed that apples, oranges, broccoli, and tomatoes would be on the list.

But it wasn't until she eliminated those foods, as well as many others, that she was cured of the eczema for the first time in her life and helped tremendously with her asthma. "Once I began eliminating the foods, my system cleared up, and I was able to identify exactly which foods were triggering the asthma," she explains. "Now, I can't even go near a jar of peanut butter without my lungs getting congested."

Food intolerance is a promising therapy for the millions . . . who long to breathe easier once again.

Christian Mayer (see "World Class Health" in chapter 1) is also among the benefactors of the attention given to the relationship between food intolerance and respiratory problems. This world-class Austrian skier, who won the World Cup in the Giant Slalom two years in a row and a bronze medal at the Winter Olympics in Lillehammer, suffered every season with breathing problems. The stuffy air in airplanes and hotels exacerbated his condition when he had to travel to competitions. Needless to say, his coach was not happy about having one of his top skiers waylaid by a health problem. He sent Christian to an Austrian physician, Dr. Stephen Shimpf, who specializes in immunotherapy and preventative medicine in Salzburg.

As he does many of his patients, Dr. Shimpf tested Christian for food intolerance using the ALCAT Test. The results of the blood test showed that the skier was intolerant to rice, milk products, wheat, apples, bananas, and beer, most of which he consumed every day. Once he removed those foods his stuffy nose cleared up. In addition, he was able to avoid (unlike some of his team members) the usual seasonal colds and flu. As an added bonus he lost the extra ten pounds he typically gained in the off-season and he had more energy. But this world-class athlete says the most important benefit is this: "I'm winning. Right after the test I won my first World Cup in America. I was surprised by the test results because I'd always thought foods like apples and bananas are healthy, but they're not for me. I avoid my reactive foods and I feel better."

Dr. Shimpf, however, was not surprised by the results. "I've gotten used to great results with food intolerance testing with my patients, so amazing results like this no longer astonish me." He has found food intolerance testing to be a big help in treating patients who suffer from respiratory conditions among other problems. Besides Christian, Dr. Shimpf points to a particularly "interesting case" of a 30-year-old woman who had endured severe asthma for years. After he tested her blood and she eliminated her reactive foods for three to four months, she was able to significantly reduce her intake of cortisone, which she'd been taking for years to deal with debilitating asthma attacks. "This reduction of intake of a pharmaceutical as strong as cortisone alone had an additional positive impact on her health," notes Schimpf.

A Promising Treatment for Millions

Many other respiratory sufferers around the world have duplicated the improvement of Moselle, Christian, and Patricia—thanks to eliminating intolerant foods from their diets. Several research studies have also shown that food does indeed have a significant impact on airway conditions. These findings clearly show a promising treatment for the millions around the world who long to breathe free once again.

Among the many interesting research results on the effects of food intolerance and respiratory health problems are the findings of two studies conducted by Drs. Peter Fell and Jonathan Brostoff. Both studies are based on the results of testing people for food intolerance using the ALCAT Test. In the first study, conducted in 1988, Drs. Fell and Brostoff reported that all eight patients who had suffered for more than three years with hay fever were successful in reducing or eliminating their upper respiratory symptoms. The researchers reported that although many of these patients were skeptical that their condition had a dietary cause, the results were clear-cut improvements due to the elimination of reactive foods. By sticking to their ALCAT-designed diets, patients maintained positive results through their follow-up exams.

In a second study conducted in 1990, Drs. Fell and Brostoff found slightly less dramatic results for patients with asthma and rhinitis, but nonetheless significant to the many people seeking non-pharmaceutical treatments to their chronic upper airways diseases. Of the patients studied, whose symptoms included sneezing, running noses, coughing, wheezing, and headaches, four of the 17 completely improved and maintained their improvement with a change in diet and only an occasional need for an accompanying treatment such as a medication or inhalers. The study's authors note that these results are not surprising considering that inhalant allergens also play a major role in these conditions.

Dr. Solomon also found mixed, but overall hopeful, results in her study of 172 patients with 11 different conditions. Among them were 20 patients with recurrent sinusitis, 108 patients with hay fever, and 18 patients with asthma. All the patients were put on diets that eliminated their allergenic foods. Within a ten-month period, Dr. Solomon found that with diet alone, 59 percent of the people with recurrent sinusitis improved, 42 percent of the patients with hay fever improved, and 30 percent of the patients with asthma improved.

Many other studies have found that food allergy is an important cause of asthma and hay fever. Among them are two relatively recent studies, including one in 1987 by Zdenek Pelikan, director of the Department of Allergy and Immunology at the Institute of Medical Sciences in the Netherlands. Pelikan investigated the role of food allergy in patients with rhinitis, some of whom had accompanying symptoms of sinusitis and headache. He found that the role of foods was confirmed in two-thirds of the patients with hay fever where an allergic component was suspected. Further, in 19 percent of these cases, food was found to be the sole cause of the patients' hay fever. In half these patients, the hay fever was caused by various inhalant allergens with foods also having an effect (known as "secondary" food allergy). Pelikan commented that "the role of food allergy and of food in general in subjects with allergic disorders, especially in those suffering from rhinitis, otitis media, and sinusitis, is still underestimated by clinicians."

In the second study, Dr. D.G. Wraith, consultant physician with the Allergy Clinic in London, tested several aspects of food intolerance in a number of patients with asthma in 1987 and concluded that "food allergy is very important cause of asthma but is often overlooked." Further, he reported, "Avoidance of the cause would prevent much disability and also lessen the amount of drugs needed, which is important considering their expense and potential side-effects."

These studies are just a few of the many going back several decades that clearly point to the relationship of food intolerance to respiratory conditions, including food intolerance in children as young as newborns. For example, Dr. Gerrard found a clear relationship between cow's milk and infants in two of his studies, entitled "Food-Induced Respiratory Disease" and "Familial Recurrent Rhinorrhea and Bronchitis Due to Cow's Milk," conducted in 1966.

Hope for a Healthy Future

The dramatically high number of respiratory sufferers is not surprising considering the complex and sensitive respiratory system. It includes miles of air passages in the lungs. By the time air reaches these passages, it has already been warmed and moistened by the nose, filtered through nose hairs and lymph tissue in the throat, and then re-filtered by millions of tiny cilia (hair-like projections along membranous cell tissue) to remove any particles that could damage the lungs.

Unfortunately for Stacey, this complex respiratory system broke down so severely that she had to have one lung removed. A downward spiral in her health quickly followed lung cancer surgery. Stacey developed pneumonia in her other lung and couldn't speak above a whisper and without extreme effort for nearly a year. She began seeing any medical practitioner who would give her any bit of hope. A chiropractor she was seeing recommended a dietitian who worked extensively in the area of food intolerance. The dietitian immediately had Stacey tested for food allergies using the ALCAT blood test. "The test was terrific," says Stacey. "It showed me the foods I was allergic to, and the minute I started eating only what the test indicated was safe for me to eat, I was able to speak without gasping for air. I speak beautifully now."

Like Patricia, Stacey showed intolerance to a long list of foods that she never would have suspected without a specific test. She can no longer eat many vegetables she used to enjoy, including everything *but* spinach, broccoli, green beans, and cabbage. She's also not able to eat condiments such as garlic, oregano, vanilla, and cinnamon. "Those are things I never would have guessed in a million years that my body couldn't tolerate. And without the test, I never would have believed that the vegetables I loved so much were killing me. Ironically, other doctors had told me to eat healthier, including eating all the vegetables I wanted. They didn't have a clue that those vegetables were helping to make me sick. I am so grateful for this test."

Stacey is among a growing number of people who were victims of inhalant allergies for years before finding a doctor who was experienced in finding the source of respiratory problems by testing a patient's blood against a battery of food allergens. The ALCAT Test also tests for sensitivities to molds and chemicals such as preservatives and food dyes—all of which can contribute either directly or indirectly to respiratory difficulties. As many practitioners believe, these intolerances represent more load on the body, and the air passages are a likely target for a system weakened by the elements.

CHAPTER 11

Skin and Food Intolerance

Imagine being completely uncomfortable in your own skin. That is a fact of life for millions who suffer from skin conditions such as eczema, urticaria, angioedema, and severe acne. Yet much of the suffering due to these puzzling skin conditions could be prevented through elimination of reactive foods. Even cellulite, the scourge of women everywhere, is closely associated with food intolerance.

Eczema and Food Sensitivities

It's a fact of life for people like Patricia, who at 26 had suffered for years with raw patches of itchy, blistered eczema from head to toe. (Patricia also suffered from asthma—see previous chapter.) Eczema, one of the most common skin conditions, is an inflammation of the outer layer of skin which, in the early stages, may be red, blistered, swollen, weeping, and extremely itchy. Later, usually after much scratching by the sufferer, it becomes crusted, scaly, and thickened. Patricia's skin was so sensitive that she had many sleepless nights. Everything irritated her raw skin, including the blankets, sheets, pillows, and pajamas. During the day her clothes irritated her skin.

Finally, the unbearable pain forced her to quit her job. After years of suffering and trying all kinds of therapies recommended by a variety of doctors, hopeless and in pain, she ended up at allergy and immunology specialist Dr. John Gerrard's office in Saskatchewan, Canada. He saw that she was a good candidate for food intolerance, since her eczema had gone away during a period when she had pneumonia and couldn't eat. The ALCAT Test identified so many reactive foods that she was left to eat only a few vegetables, a few fruits, and some organically raised meat. As soon as she eliminated her reactive foods, her eczema cleared up right away. "Without this test I would have never known foods were aggravating my eczema. This test identified which foods bothered me."

Virginia, another person suffering from eczema, says that since childhood she'd had problems with allergies and eczema, and that when she was 18, the eczema suddenly got worse, then went downhill from there. With her first pregnancy, her skin "went totally wild." Her diet is so limited now that she has to be very careful with her meals. She eats seasonal foods as much as possible and rotates the foods to which she has no sensitivity. Whenever she grows lax with her meals, she immediately starts itching again. "Even one bite of apple makes me itchy. And if I eat beef my skin gets raw."

Virginia's story is not the only extreme case of a skin condition that responded well to food intolerance testing. Thousands of patients—both adults and children—are enjoying healthy skin, free of irritations, by eliminating foods to which they showed intolerance. However, while traditional medicine recognizes food allergy if the result is an *immediate* skin rash, when the reaction is delayed, as it often is in food intolerance, traditional doctors tend to ignore the possibility of food sensitivity as a cause of the skin problems. This is true despite success stories like Virginia's and many research studies by respected medical professionals. "Early in my career I learned that careful dietary histories are important in treating patients and that ordinary, healthy foods can cause many problems, including skin conditions," says Dr. Gerrard, former professor of Pediatrics at the University of Saskatchewan, Canada. He has conducted a great deal of research on the topic. "It's a great disappointment that doctors just don't bother to consider food intolerance, because foods can be so helpful with so many different problems."

Itching to Be Allergic

"Many controversies exist about the nature and importance of adverse reactions to food and chemical additives to human diseases, and the whole spectrum of symptoms that may appear are not delineated," explains Lene Høj, a Danish doctor of internal medicine and specialist in allergic diseases. "But my success in treating patients and my research in the area of food intolerance clearly shows that a long list of conditions and symptoms are related to food allergies including eczema and urticaria." One of the most severe skin conditions that Dr. Høj has seen in her 17 years in practice as an allergy specialist in Denmark was a four-year-old boy named Henry, whose skin was so covered in rashes, scars, and wounds that he was tormented day and night by itching. It seemed that no matter what Henry's mother tried, her son's condition only got worse.

His suffering began when his mother stopped breast-feeding him and put him on commercial formula. An itching rash began appearing on his face and arms, and his constant scratching left the skin raw and bloody. When his mother put gloves on his hands to try and prevent him from scratching his wounds, he would rub his skin against carpets and on furniture. He looked so different from other children his age that he became withdrawn, developed learning disabilities, and began having suicidal thoughts. After seeing a battery of doctors, Henry was using six types of allergy medications and a special skin cream, which did little to ease his physical pain.

Dr. Høj tested him for food and chemical sensitivities using the ALCAT Test and found Henry had many allergies. His mother began carefully preparing his daily meals, which consisted of lowfat yogurt without sugar for breakfast, and whole-grain rye bread and ham, tuna fish, or specially made liver paté without bacon for lunch. Finally, his condition was under control, his skin cleared up, and Henry began picking up where his life left off. The condition took its toll psychologically, but today he goes to school with other children who have developmental problems. He now has a job, but has to wear special gloves so that his skin is protected from irritants like dust. Henry's mother doesn't mind the daily preparation of food, which includes making all the meals from scratch. She's just glad that her son is able to live a somewhat normal life.

With regards to food allergy and skin conditions, Høj explains that when allergy is the root of eczema and urticaria, the mast cells in the lower layers of the skin are believed to cause the problem. When they degranulate, the mediators that are released have a powerful effect on the capillaries (tiny blood vessels) that lie all around them in the skin. These capillaries become leakier, allowing plasma (the watery part of the blood) to seep out into the skin itself. This produces the characteristic swellings and itchiness of urticaria, which is a skin disruption with temporary welts of various shapes and sizes with clear margins and pale centers. Urticaria is often thought to be triggered by food, drugs, and stress. Sometimes it's triggered by cold. Where a great deal of seepage from the blood vessels occurs, the tissues below the skin may also become filled with watery fluid. This produces a puffiness that doctors describe as localized angioedema (or edema), an abnormal pooling of fluid in the tissues.

A Child's Pain Is Everyone's Pain

When a child is in pain, parents suffer as much or more than the child does. So you can imagine their relief to find a correct diagnosis of food intolerance after years of futile medical treatments. A mother in Germany wrote to Mr. Just Hintz, laboratory manager in Hamburg, Germany, after finally finding the solution to her daughter's suffering:

> I am sending a few lines to express my thanks and appreciation to you. No doctor was able to help my daughter, who suffered severely from neurodermatitis. In June 1990, we came to your office the first time. Sarah, who was born in February 1985, was six months old when she developed red, itchy skin. After seeing several doctors, she was diagnosed with neurodermatitis, and treated for five years with cortisone cream. These creams did not bring about any healing, only some short-term relief.
>
> In the meantime, the disease had increased to the point that our whole family was suffering, both physically and psychologically. No one could get a good night's sleep; we felt sick right along with Sarah. She lived with a constant, strong urge to scratch, and whenever she scratched her whole body would be full of scabs and open wounds. She had all of the classic symptoms, which are very well known to the medical community. But what is not well

known is the method you used to treat her condition. When she was tested for food intolerance in June 1990, we were told with great astonishment the foods that Sarah is reacting to allergically. At the beginning, we were shocked, wondering how we could handle all of this. Her whole diet had to be changed, including no more rye and sugar; several spices and vegetables had to go away if we wanted to have success. Now, three years later we are so happy that all these efforts have paid off. Her new diet was a complete success for every one of us, but mainly for Sarah, who had suffered for so long. Seeing her perfectly smooth skin now, it seems like a miracle.

Hives and Food Intolerance

In traditional medicine, skin rashes such as eczema and urticaria are believed to be predominantly a problem among children. But as Virginia's and others' stories point out, adults are not excepted from these conditions. Shortly after starting a new job as a banker in the fall of 1995, Frank came down with bronchitis. Knowing he was allergic to penicillin, his doctors put him on another antibiotic. He woke up just days later with hives all over his body and big painful blisters on his face and head. His doctor diagnosed urticaria.

No matter what Frank tried or what his doctors prescribed, the hives didn't go away or even improve. Finally, at the suggestion of a co-worker, he made an appointment with Dr. Barbara Solomon. After listening to his medical history, she recommended an ALCAT Test. He showed intolerance to several foods including sugar, wheat, corn, pork, and some fish. After eliminating those foods, as best as he could in his busy career as a banker, his condition improved to a manageable level.

Ironically, shortly after that, his wife was hospitalized for a heart condition. Her second day in the hospital, Patsy broke out in a rash and was swollen from head to toe. "I was one big, swollen sore all over my body." Her family doctor diagnosed angioedema. Many conditions can cause angioedema, such as heart or kidney failure and allergic reactions. He thought that it was an allergy to something, but never guessed that the food she was given in the hospital was the cause. Dr. Solomon tested her and found allergies to several foods, including chicken, potatoes, and green beans—the very foods she'd been fed in the hospital the night before her skin broke out. By eliminating their intolerant foods, she and her husband were able to get relief from the hives and blisters, as well as improve their overall health and lose several pounds of excess weight.

Acne Relief with Food Elimination

Allergy testing is not just for severe skin conditions. Many people have had success at clearing up acne, especially as a side effect of eliminating intolerant foods for other medical conditions. Brenda, a banker in her early 40s, for example, had an ALCAT Test done to improve her overall health. She had few food intolerances, but one of her primary sensitivities was to cinnamon. After eliminating the spice, her chronic acne cleared up completely.

As shown with these patient case histories, there is no effective way to diagnose food intolerance for each person without individual testing. Guesswork alone will not help most people find out which foods, chemicals, and other substances they should not eat. While one person can eat chicken, like Patsy's husband, others such as

Patsy herself cannot. One person, like Henry, can eat rye but not wheat; another, like Sarah, breaks out if she eats rye. Despite success stories like these, you'll find few traditional allergy doctors who would agree that delayed food reactions cause skin conditions.

One of the problems in their lack of acceptance of this therapy is that many current research studies on food intolerance and skin conditions show just over 50 percent improvement—which many do not believe is statistically significant. These studies may not show results as high as those of other studies on food intolerance and conditions such as migraine, fatigue, and weight loss. But 50 percent improvement does show nonetheless that food intolerance is clearly a viable therapy for at least half of the millions of people who suffer from painful skin irritations. It means that the Virginias, Franks, Sarahs, and Patsys in the world get their chance to live a pain-free life.

In several research studies on the ALCAT Test, doctors found over 50 percent improvement in eczema, urticaria, angioedema, and general skin condition by eliminating specific food intolerances. In their 1988 study on the ALCAT Test, Drs. Fell and Brostoff found that patients with eczema and urticaria who stuck to their ALCAT diets improved over a six-week period. In a second study in 1990 on the effectiveness of the ALCAT Test in treating four common patient complaints, Drs. Fell and Brostoff found that after one year 26 patients (9 with urticaria and 17 with eczema) improved by an estimated 50 percent. The nine urticaria patients showed a striking improvement—two completely resolved and six maintained their success rate over the course of the 12-month study.

Consistent with this percentage, Dr. Barbara Solomon reported in 1992 that 11 patients with eczema improved by 55 percent when they eliminated their intolerant foods.

Further, Dr. J. R. Cabo-Soler, M.D., a medical faculty member and chief of the Biochemistry Department at the University of Valencia in Spain, noted that in addition to losing weight, patients also reported greater quality to their skin—more smoothness and less dryness and flaking,

Eczema Improves with Weight Loss

In a one-month study on the relationship of food intolerance to weight loss, body composition, and self-reported disease symptoms conducted in 1995 at the Columbia/ HCA Medical Center's Sports Medicine and Performance Center in Houston, lead investigator Gilbert Kaats, Ph.D., found a much higher than 50 percent improvement in eczema symptoms after patients followed a diet that eliminated their intolerant foods. In fact, the individuals in the experimental group (50 participants) who had reported problems with eczema averaged a 66 percent improvement in their skin condition after following the diet.

On the other hand, those in the control group (50 individuals) who reported eczema problems said that their skin condition got about 33 percent *worse* after following diets of their own choosing. Interestingly, both groups reported nearly the same level of skin trouble at the beginning of study. "While the individuals on the ALCAT diet consistently performed better than the control group in all disease-symptom categories, eczema was the only condition in which the control group actually reported *worse* symptoms while on diets of their own choosing," said Dr. Kaats, director of the Health and Medical Research Foundation, an independent research organization in San Antonio.

Reactive Foods Get under Your Skin

For the past several decades many researchers from around the world, all known for their special interest in atopic eczema, have independently described the value of food intolerance as a therapy for chronic skin conditions. Among them, Dr. Alfred Rowe in 1951 found a correlation between food allergies and atopic dermatitis in infants and children. In 1966, Dr. G. Hagerman examined the importance of food factors in atopic dermatitis. In 1978, Dr. P. Juto found a strict elimination diet effective in the treatment of infantile atopic eczema. Michael Pike, Research Fellow, Institute of Child Health, London, found a measurable improvement in skin problems using elimination diets. He said:

> These data do provide evidence that, in at least some individuals with atopic eczema, ingestion of certain foods will provoke a reaction of some kind, be it eczematous or urticaria. We are often asked by skeptical [sic] colleagues, "Do you really believe all this 'food business'?" It remains one of the sadder aspects of mainstream medicine that we should see such an important problem as a question of "belief" or "non-belief." What is actually needed is an open, inquiring attitude, and careful, critical investigation. By failing to study the relationship between foods and atopic eczema, we might deny ourselves the opportunity of understanding and thus eventually overcoming this common and distressing disease.

Medical experts who recognize food intolerance believe in this therapy as an effective option for many skin condition sufferers. "There is growing evidence that what goes into the mouth can produce a reaction in the skin, and that food is an important factor," says Dr. Brostoff.

Dr. Stephen Schimpf, the preventive medicine and immunotherapy doctor who treated Austria's Olympic skiers, said that by eliminating intolerant foods, in accordance with test results, one patient with severe psoriasis was cured of all his allergic-like symptoms including severe itching and skin so hot at night that he couldn't sleep. "Now he's able to get a good night's sleep. We've seen many patients' allergic-like symptoms go away when they eliminate their allergenic foods."

Dr. I. A. Schapkaitz, a general practitioner in Johannesburg, South Africa, found the ALCAT Test a great help in his practice, in particular with eczema and urticaria. "When you've had a patient with severe urticaria who has suffered for months on end, and you put them on an ALCAT diet and see them get better, as a physician it's very gratifying and rewarding."

Cellulite—Such a Pretty Name

No discussion of fat or overweight would be complete without some reference to cellulite. This anatomical eyesore, which very much affects the appearance of skin, has become the dread of every woman in a bathing suit. So poorly understood, and yet so hated, cellulite is the result of modern lifestyles to a great extent. According to Dr. Elizabeth Dancey in her book *The Cellulite Solution,* "95% of women have or believe they have cellulite."

It is hard to believe that there is as yet no known cure for a condition that affects such a large segment of the population. Since no established medical treatment protocol exists, most physicians avoid treating cellulite. This opens the way for any number of unscrupulous purveyors of potions to make their pitch to a captive audience of sufferers. To opportunistic entrepreneurs, *cellulite* means "sell you a lot." Interestingly, these potions are not held to the same demanding standards as drugs since they are not applied as a medical intervention. Sales are soaring.

Cellulite is found only in fatty tissue (no one has ever had cellulite in muscle or bone!). But one does not have to be overweight to have cellulite. Cellulite in women most frequently appears on the hips, buttocks, and thighs. Men will tend to develop cellulite on the upper body.

Even cellulite, the scourge of women everywhere, is associated with food intolerance.

Fat storage in the body is controlled by special receptors in each fat cell. These receptors are called alpha2 receptors. Various hormones may stimulate alpha2 receptors and open the doors into the fat cell to allow the deposit of more fat into the cell. The most prominent of these hormones is insulin. Insulin in the blood encourages more fat to be deposited into storage.

On the other hand, beta-receptors open the figurative back door of the fat cells to allow fat out into the bloodstream. Hormones that stimulate the beta-receptors are thyroxin and adrenaline.

As Dr. Dancey poignantly points out in her book, "not all fat is created equal." In women the fat cells around the hips, thighs, and buttocks have six times as many alpha2 receptors as beta-receptors. This implies that fat can be stored six times as fast as it can be released from these areas. Many women will attest to this truth. Elsewhere in the body there are six times as many beta-receptors as alpha2 receptors. This means fat will be lost six times as fast from these areas. Therefore, physiologically, if fat is to be gained, it will most likely show in the hips, thighs, and buttocks. And when fat is lost, it will come from the upper body in most women. This is truly the worst of both worlds and explains a lot. No matter the reason for the weight gain, the overweight will appear on the hips, thighs, and buttocks of most women and on the upper body on men.

Most important to the issues discussed in this book is the high incidence of cellulite in individuals with food intolerance. It seems that food intolerance and its resultant fluid retention, caused by immune-mediated damage to blood vessels, may be a significant contributor to the appearance of cellulite. Those who successfully identify and treat food intolerance may notice an improvement in cellulite. Likewise, quite often those with cellulite may suspect food intolerance. Cellulite may be prevented by the prompt elimination of food intolerance, improvement of lymphatic drainage, and the regeneration of blood supply to these areas of compromised blood supply.

Cellulite actually describes fatty tissue in various stages of development. The word *cellulite* refers to the dimpling appearance of the skin associated with the more advanced stages of change in the subcutaneous fat. Although areas of advanced and long-standing fatty deterioration may be irreparable, much cellulite is actually tissue in a dynamic state of evolution. The latter is amenable to revitalization.

Treatment of cellulite begins with the reversal of adverse physiological changes that predispose to the deterioration of subcutaneous fat. Once the evolution of cellulite is halted, attention may turn to the reversal of body physiology that sustains existing cellulitic tissue. Remember that fatty tissue by its nature and purpose is in a continual state of active change. Successful control of the appearance of cellulite will require ongoing attention to avoiding the negative lifestyle factors that predispose cellulite. A thorough cellulite treatment program will include identification and elimination of food intolerance. Until intolerant foods are eliminated, any improvement in cellulite appearance will be temporary, as cellulite will continue to develop due to deterioration of the circulation in these fatty areas. Once the food sensitivities are eliminated, special efforts to improve circulation and lymphatic drainage in these areas may proceed. The most effective maintenance of healthy tissue appearance is achieved through healthy eating habits:

- **Avoid processed and packaged foods.** These foods are stripped of nutrient value and filled with chemicals to prolong shelf life. They are often rich in simple carbohydrates and fats and tend to cause insulin levels to soar. This results in prompt storing of the empty fat calories as fat on your body. (Remember, they are six times more likely to be stored as fat in the hips, thighs, and buttocks in women.)

- **Drink at least two and preferably three quarts of fresh water each day.** This should be filtered or bottled spring water to avoid the unpleasant effects of large doses of chlorine on the intestinal bacteria. Also, a fairly large number of people, especially asthmatics, are sensitive to chlorine.

- **Limit caffeine.** Two cups of coffee per day should be the limit. You may also be sensitive to caffeine, however.

- **Avoid alcoholic beverages.** Notwithstanding their possible beneficial effect on heart function when consumed in moderation, these empty calories are destined for your fat bank, which ironically is a strain on your heart.

- **Avoid foods with high salt content.** These foods promote fluid retention and contribute to cellulite.

Some other helpful suggestions in addition to eating tips include:

- **Establish a daily lower body aerobic exercise routine.** This would ideally include getting up from sitting every hour or two and moving around. Routine contraction of the leg muscles prevents pooling of venous and lymphatic drainage.
- **Avoid wearing tight-fitting clothing, especially around the waist and thighs.** Compression of the lymphatic drainage at these points promotes accumulation of fluid in the fatty tissue of the buttocks, hips, and thighs. Pantyhose may be the biggest culprit here.
- **Avoid sitting and/or crossing the legs for long periods of time.** Get up and move around frequently to improve blood flow and circulation to the lower body. This allows the removal of accumulated toxins from these tissues and improves oxygenation of healthy cells.
- **Consider lymphatic drainage and cellulite massage.** We use the *Lipotherapie* technique in our office with very favorable results. This technique makes use of a therapeutic massage machine, which utilizes a combination of variable suction pressures along with mechanical rolling of the tissue. The massage seems to improve the healthy appearance of the skin as it contours and shapes the cellulitic areas. This procedure is also complementary to weight loss, as it tones loose skin and stimulates blood flow. Although no mechanical device

will substitute for healthy habits and skills, Lipotherapie has turned out to be a resourceful modality when
life's pressures preclude a comprehensive cellulite prevention program.

- **Practice deep-breathing exercises several times a day.**
  This practice is a healthy way to stimulate lymphatic
  flow from the pelvis to the chest where it enters the
  bloodstream.
- **Perform a gentle brushing of the areas of cellulite on
  a daily basis.** This is best done with a soft brush using
  very gentle strokes across the affected areas. Stroking
  toward the heart stimulates lymphatic drainage in the
  proper direction.

Cellulite may be viewed as a continuation of the effects of food intolerance. As we have established earlier
in this book, food intolerance can make you fat. Now we
understand that food intolerance, if not eliminated, will
make existing fat deposits even more unsightly. Find out
and eliminate your reactive foods.

CHAPTER 12

Fatigue and Food Intolerance

"My goodness, is it really that simple, Doctor? After all those years of seeing so many doctors and spending hundreds of dollars in supplements, then, just by not eating my allergenic foods, my fatigue is completely gone."

That comment is from Cheryl, a woman in her mid-30s who had suffered for years with chronic fatigue. In early 1990, she went to see Dr. David Cafarelli at the suggestion of a friend. After years of trying many different therapies to rid her of the constant fatigue that plagued her life, she'd nearly given up hope that any doctor could help her. As soon as she described her medical history to Dr. Cafarelli, he tested her for food intolerance; sure enough, she was sensitive to several foods including three she was eating nearly every day—tomatoes, potatoes, and eggplant.

Dr. Cafarelli, a medical practitioner in West Palm Beach for the past 14 years, sees many people with chronic illnesses, including fatigue, who've tried every-thing and can't get well. Nutritional treatments are a big part of his therapy, including testing for food intolerance using the ALCAT Test. "I go by the motto that anything as fundamental as eating is imperative to look at before you move on and get fancy with other tests and treat-ments," he says. "When a person has food intolerance, which I believe includes nearly everyone, I'm able to find the offending foods right away with this test."

Fatigue: An Early Warning

Fatigue is a common feature of many diseases and ill-nesses. Evidence implicates food intolerance as a cause of fatigue and even suggests that fatigue may be an "early warning sign" of food intolerance.

Dr. Paul Jaconello, a nutritional and preventative medicine specialist in Ontario, Canada, also believes that food is a fundamental part of a complete medical diagno-sis, particularly in the area of chronic fatigue. "Certain foods in certain people can trigger a 'biochemical cas-cade.' Once the body is overloaded, these reactions can manifest as excessive fatigue or they can manifest in any organ of the body, or both." One of his patients, named Jamie, had reached a point of overload while dealing with her mother's death due to lung cancer.

The death was a wake-up call to address her own health, and in her grief she tried to give up smoking. But 38 years of not watching her diet, combined with the stress of her mother's death, overloaded her system; her cholesterol level skyrocketed and she started gaining weight. A conventional high-carbohydrate diet, pre-scribed by a dietitian to address Jamie's high cholesterol, left her feeling lethargic, and she started retaining water.

Dr. Jaconello suggested that eliminating her food intolerances might help. The ALCAT Test showed her intolerant to common foods like wheat, broccoli, potatoes, grapefruit, and oranges. Not long after removing these foods from her diet, her cholesterol level returned to normal range, her energy level and mental clarity climbed, and the water retention was significantly reduced.

Fatigue may be an "early warning sign" of food intolerance.

Cindy, another fatigue sufferer, also decided that something wasn't right after she finally lost weight on a popular diet. The diet left her feeling constantly hungry, fatigued, and cold. The ALCAT Test, prescribed by Dr. Richard Bahr, a specialist in environmental medicine in Cincinnati, showed her to be allergic to several foods including soybeans, zucchini, tomatoes, wheat, and tuna. She said that she ate soybeans, zucchini, and tomatoes often. She strictly followed the prescribed rotation diet and the tiredness was gone. "I was amazed at how much more energy I had," she said. "When we identify their major food intolerances, the patients usually respond rather well," notes Dr. Bahr.

Cheryl, Jamie, and Cindy's stories are not unusual. Like so many others with serious medical conditions, many people have been cured of fatigue—including low energy and chronic fatigue syndrome—by eliminating the foods to which they showed intolerance. Normally, people experience fatigue after they've exerted a great deal of energy. However, if their tiredness is not related to any particular exertion on their part, is unrelieved by rest or sleep, and is frequently worse in the morning, many health practitioners believe it is probably associated in some way with food and/or chemical sensitivities. Persistent fatigue, while not necessarily life-threatening, can be a debilitating, life-wrecking medical condition, severely limiting a person's potential, both personally and professionally. Yet it is widespread and appears, like many medical conditions due to food intolerance, to be growing.

Most experts find fatigue so common that putting a number on how many people suffer from excessive tiredness is impossible. According to a *Health* magazine report (October 1995), "One in four Americans have fatigue lasting longer than two weeks, often beyond six months." In a May 14, 1979, issue of *U.S. News and World Report,* Dr. John E. Bulette, a psychiatrist at the Medical College of Pennsylvania, stated that 50 percent of all patients admitted to general hospitals in the U.S. list fatigue as a major complaint. According to Dr. Theron Randolph, in *An Alternative Approach to Allergies,* "One of the most commonly occurring symptoms in medicine, and especially in the histories of allergy patients, is chronic fatigue. Although fatigue may be the only manifestation of their problem, it more commonly exists in conjunction with other manifestations."

While many people are like Cheryl, Jamie, and Cindy, for whom fatigue is the dominant symptom, another category of patients exists for whom fatigue is a secondary symptom that accompanies a major symptom, and which can also be helped by addressing food allergy. In fact it's not unusual for ALCAT patients with any condition, such as obesity, irritable bowel, or migraines, to remark, "I have so much more energy," after removing their intolerant foods.

Christine, for example, was so "bone weary" in 1990 that she couldn't put one foot in front of the other, even though she slept all night long. For several months prior to the onset of her severe fatigue, her health had been deteriorating. In particular, she was experiencing increasingly severe chest pains and heart palpitations, and she had muscle aches in her arms. Finally, her condition landed her in the hospital. While there, she became even more tired and achy. Two days after she returned home, she was back in the hospital with severe chest pains and a rash that had developed all over her body. Her doctors were mystified by her condition; try as they might, they couldn't find the source of her mounting problems.

When she left the hospital for the second time, she immediately made an appointment with Dr. Barbara Solomon, an internal medicine physician who specializes in alternative therapies in Maryland. Dr. Solomon had successfully treated Christine's husband for a chronic, debilitating skin rash by locating his food intolerances. Dr. Solomon had an ALCAT Test completed on Christine. As soon as Christine stopped eating her reactive foods, she felt better. "It was unbelievable. From the very day I stopped eating my intolerant foods I started getting better. The tiredness lifted, the chest pains subsided, and the rash disappeared. My primary care physician couldn't believe how fast I improved. Also, I learned that the reason I had felt so much worse in the hospital was the food they fed me, like chicken, potatoes, and green beans, all of which I am highly reactive to."

Few people will respond as quickly as Christine did, but her story dramatically illustrates the fact that traditional medical practices rarely recognize food intolerance, even when it's right under their noses, as it was when Patsy was in the hospital. I have been impressed with the number of patients in my own practice who relate how much more energetic they feel after the first week away from their reactive foods.

More Common Than You'd Think

Even though it's so common, fatigue almost seems to not be considered a serious medical condition by the general medical community. Even the debilitating disease known as chronic fatigue syndrome gets short shrift by most doctors. An article in *Newsweek* in April 1996 reported that, "There is no question the health establishment has erred on the side of complacency." As a result, many people with hidden food allergies that manifest as fatigue, and other symptoms, go to doctor after doctor seeking relief.

Denise, for example, is the kind of patient whom doctors derogatorily refer to as hypochondriacs or as having "thick file syndrome" because they go to doctors so often complaining about so many different symptoms. Denise went from one doctor to another for nine years complaining of fatigue, sore muscles, a painful knot in her shoulder, depression, sinus problems, overweight, and insomnia. While she would insist that something was wrong with her, the doctors would make comments such as "You're just stressed because you're a busy mom" or the classic "It's all in your head." When she was 56 pounds overweight, one doctor prescribed diet pills. "I had more energy, but they sped me up so much that I dumped them in the toilet. The last thing I needed, on top of everything else, was to become addicted to drugs."

She never got any relief from any of her symptoms until she went to see Dr. Anthony Ferro in West Chester, Pennsylvania. He diagnosed food intolerance and prescribed an ALCAT Test. Denise was intolerant to a long list of foods including wheat, potatoes, sugar, dairy products, and several vegetables. She'd been eating these in salads nearly every day as prescribed by various weight-loss diets. By modifying her diet she immediately lost weight and the fatigue lifted, as did all her other symptoms. "I had felt like I was on the road to death, spinning out of control. I was surprised to find that I had any food allergies, let alone so many. I was very pleased to find the solution as simple as food allergies, because if I'd stayed on a low-calorie diet and prescription drugs I would be much worse off today."

Many people like Denise feel that their lives were literally rescued by finding out that allergenic foods were making them sick and tired. A popular opera singer in Denmark was living a celebrity's pampered lifestyle, including eating the best food and drinking the best wine that money could buy, until the day he collapsed on stage. Just prior to his collapse, the Royal Opera House was being renovated and dust was everywhere. Suddenly, one night while performing, his throat closed, his eyes burned, and he became so tired he had to be carried off the stage. After that episode he couldn't return to the stage, due to both his fear and to his extreme exhaustion.

Terrified for his health and his career, he traveled to the U.S. to see one of the leading allergy experts; ironically, it wasn't until he returned to Denmark and was referred to Dr. Lene Høj, a Danish allergist in Copenhagen, that he got relief. She tested him for food and chemical allergies and found several of both, including calves' liver, which he was so reactive to that it was "pure poison" for him. He went on a strict diet and had his home cleared of all chemicals. He became a discriminating eater at parties and brought his own sulfite-free wine when socializing. Within a short time he was able to return to the stage.

The opera singer's experience is one of many classic stories which help confirm the belief of many environmental and preventative health physicians—that one reason a food intolerance manifests is because the body reaches a state of overload. This performer had been eating all the wrong foods, drinking the wrong beverages, and living with toxins that were depressing his body's immune system. His daily exposure to a new allergen—dust—was the proverbial straw that broke the camel's back and he could no longer continue taxing his system with the toxins in certain foods and chemicals.

Trail Benedict believes that his and his father's systems were overloaded from working in the family's chemical laboratory business, where they handled many pesticides. Both suffered from extreme fatigue—Trail to the point that he was falling asleep while driving to work, despite getting a good night's sleep every night. His family switched to the nutritional supplement business in the early 1980s, but none of the supplements they sold to others for improving health gave them more energy. Finally, Trail and his father learned about the ALCAT Test. Once they eliminated their allergenic foods, both had more energy than they'd had in years. Trail also lost 20 pounds he'd wanted to shed. "Eliminating our allergenic foods had a dramatic effect on our health. I knew I had allergies but I couldn't pinpoint them. The ALCAT identified them for me."

Further Evidence Links Food to Fatigue

Patient success stories are not the only proof that food intolerance can be the culprit in fatigue and low energy. Many of the researchers, including prominent professionals in the field of food intolerance, consistently find a strong link between food allergies and fatigue. As early as 1946, Dr. Theron Randolph published studies on allergy as a causative factor in fatigue and weakness. In 1950, Dr. Albert Rowe published a paper on allergic toxemia and fatigue. And in 1954, Dr. Frederic Speer published a study on fatigue and its relationship to food allergy.

Dr. William Crook also listed fatigue as one of the systemic manifestations due to allergy in children in 1961.

Current research studies on the ALCAT Test also show that addressing food intolerance does lead to improvement in people's fatigue symptoms. One study was conducted by Dr. Solomon to determine whether the ALCAT Test was a valuable technique for physicians treating environmental illness. She studied a group of 172 patients seen in her primary care internal medicine practice for a wide range of symptoms, including fatigue, depression, migraines, gastrointestinal problems, arthritis, asthma, obesity, and eczema. Dr. Solomon reported that of the 97 cases of tension fatigue syndrome, 60 percent of the patients improved just from removing their allergenic foods from their diets. "These patients were among a category of patients who come to me as a last resort. They never suspected that foods trigger their symptoms."

One study found that the ALCAT Test has a truly predictable capacity for detecting food sensitivity. Drs. Fell and Brostoff from the Department of Immunology at the University College and Middlesex School of Medicine found that all the females in the study, aged 20 to 45, who presented with fatigue syndrome showed improvement by eliminating allergenic foods.

In a study on the relationship of food intolerance to weight loss, body composition, and self-reported disease symptoms conducted in 1994 at the Columbia/HCA Medical Center's Sports Medicine and Performance Center in Houston, lead investigator Gilbert Kaats, Ph.D., found a marked improvement in chronic tiredness, tension fatigue syndrome, lack of energy, and insomnia when sufferers eliminated their intolerant foods. While both the experimental group and control group (50 participants each) reported the same degree of chronic tiredness, the people on an individualized ALCAT diet for four weeks reported that their tiredness had improved by 50 percent. And the people who followed diets of their own choosing for four weeks reported *no* change in their chronic tiredness. Further, with tension fatigue syndrome the control group scored slightly higher than the experimental group at the beginning of the study, and at the end they scored only a marginal improvement. The people following an ALCAT diet, however, reported a 67 percent improvement. With the symptom "lack of energy," the ALCAT dieters reported just over 50 percent improvement, while the non–ALCAT dieters reported only about 10 percent improvement. With insomnia, the ALCAT dieters reported nearly 66 percent improvement at the end of the study, while the control group reported barely 5 percent improvement. "In all four categories these findings are highly statistically significant," explains Dr. Kaats, director of the Health and Medical Research Foundation, an independent research organization in San Antonio. "The chance of these results occurring at random are very slim. In other words, if you repeated the study 1,000 times, 999 times you would get the same scores for tension fatigue syndrome, and you would get the same scores 996 times for chronic tiredness and insomnia. This is a good indication that the results are not due to random chance."

Other doctors have also found success treating patients with fatigue by eliminating their sensitive foods. "Chronic fatigue patients often have underlying food sensitivities," says Dr. Jaconello. Dr. Ronald Lesko is well known in the area of metabolic problems, allergies, and chronic fatigue, and treats many patients from all over the U.S. He tests the majority of them for food intolerance using the ALCAT Test and finds the test helpful in diagnosing the cause of symptoms and in designing a dietetic program to treat the fatigue. Dr. Stephen Smith, of

Richland, Washington, says, "I treat people with chronic fatigue, and we do have success."

Even with scientific studies, patients' personal experiences, and physicians' success stories, the fact that fatigue (including chronic fatigue syndrome) can be alleviated by eliminating intolerant foods from a person's diet is not generally accepted by the medical community. But physicians who accept food intolerance believe, like Dr. Randolph, that fatigue may be the most characteristic part of food and chemical susceptibility. They believe that if no obvious medical condition, such as heart problems, chronic infection, or cancer, exist, food or chemical allergy should definitely be suspected. "The majority of allergic individuals with the fatigue syndrome have been previously diagnosed as 'neurotics,'" notes Dr. Randolph, due to physicians' typical separation of mental and physical problems. But he found that chemicals in the environment are slowly poisoning them, as their reactions to commonly eaten foods indicate. It's no wonder that patients who are chronically fatigued develop mental symptoms as well. Who wouldn't be upset if they were too exhausted to live their lives and fulfill their responsibilities?

Why So Tired?

Brostoff points out in *The Complete Guide to Food Allergy and Intolerance* that excessive tiredness can be caused by many infectious diseases, by anemia, or by an underactive thyroid gland, which can also be brought on by food intolerance. "Fatigue is very often reported as a symptom of food intolerance, especially in connection with migraines and irritable bowel syndrome. Early-morning tiredness is the most frequent problem. Looking back over case histories, it seems that fatigue may be an early warning sign as food intolerance develops." How foods might produce fatigue is not known. But Dr. Brostoff suggests that exorphines (peptides very similar to endorphins, which are natural opioids that help turn off pain in our bodies) may play a part, or it may be a side effect of some generalized immune reaction, as is suspected in post-viral syndrome.

In a great number of cases, fatigue persists following a viral infection, and this is now known as post-viral syndrome or chronic fatigue syndrome. Due to so much press, chronic fatigue syndrome is a well-known, often misdiagnosed condition. Although many people are chronically tired, true chronic fatigue syndrome is characterized by debilitating tiredness for over six months. It is accompanied by a long list of symptoms, including cognitive function problems, visual disturbances, psychological problems, shortness of breath, dizziness and balance problems, sensitivity to extreme temperatures, and chest pains, according to the Chronic Fatigue and Immune Dysfunction Syndrome Association of America (CFIDSAA).

A great deal of study has been done on chronic fatigue syndrome—which is believed to affect four to ten out of every 100,000 adults—with few, if any, conclusive answers. Beginning in the early 1990s, a growing number of researchers concluded that chronic fatigue is a serious, albeit mysterious, medical problem. Some believe it's caused by a virus, since many people come down with the syndrome soon after a flu-like illness. When you get an infection, you produce proteins called cytokines, which facilitate communication between and activate certain white blood cells, which then devour bacteria and other invaders. In addition to killing the invaders, cytokines also lay you low, and their effects can persist for some time.

Other sufferers get chronic fatigue after a psychological trauma, or a period of intense work, suggesting that stress hormones may cause it. Those who treat it as a real disease generally agree on a few basic ideas. One theory is that chronic fatigue syndrome results from a dysfunction of the immune system. A virus, stress, or another trauma somehow jump-starts the immune system, which then remains activated instead of gearing down as it would after an infection. As a result, a number of immune factors (some of which cause fatigue) remain indefinitely in high concentrations in the blood.

According to the CFIDSAA, "The exact nature of this dysfunction is not well defined," "but it can generally be viewed as an up-regulated or overactive state. Ironically, there is also evidence of some immune suppression. For example, in many patients there are functional deficiencies in natural killer cells (an important component of the immune system responsible for fighting viruses)." In other words, these patients have a compromised immune system, which is weak and at the same time hyperactive. This paradox is not uncommon. Often when an organ has to work overtime, due to some primary deficiency, it becomes enlarged. For example, the pancreas becomes enlarged when, in order to aid digestion, it is required to produce extra enzymes to compensate for the consumption of enzyme-deficient foods.

This thinking correlates with Brostoff's research in the area of fatigue and the immune system. He points out that all lymphocytes produce small messenger molecules, known as lymphokines, to communicate with each other. One important messenger molecule is interferon, whose main job is to combat viral infections. Interferon makes cells resistant to virus, but it also produces a long list of side effects such as severe fatigue, dizziness, joint pain, and headaches—symptoms remarkably similar to those of chronic fatigue syndrome. Since most cases seem to follow a viral infection of some sort, the parallel with the side effects of interferon suggests that "the immune system has overreacted to a viral infection and is continuing to produce excessive amounts of interferon. If this is the case (and there is no definitive proof that it is), then interferon might also play a role in food intolerance. Perhaps some unknown immune reaction to food stimulates the body to produce interferon, or other lymphokines, in damaging amounts. It is interesting that many chronic fatigue sufferers have been greatly helped by an elimination diet—it would seem that reactions to food are contributing to their symptoms."

Energetic Again

If this theory can be proven, it would explain Cleason's experience with chronic fatigue syndrome (see chapter 1). In December 1986, Cleason developed a bad flu. It lingered longer than usual and finally seemed to resolve. Then in March he got another flu, after which he just couldn't wake up. Constant headaches and diarrhea accompanied his daily fatigue. He dragged himself out of bed and pushed himself to go to work. Soon he started missing work. By September, the fatigue had taken its full toll and he stopped working altogether.

For all those months he saw one doctor after another with no relief. He got to the point that he lost confidence in the doctors' ability to help him. But with eight children and a wife to support, he had to try something. Finally, his wife encouraged him to have an ALCAT Test. Two of their children, one of whom was hyperactive and one who had gastrointestinal problems, had been successfully treated for food sensitivities. Cleason was tested for 100 foods, and for mold and pollen allergies. He showed a long list of sensitivities. As soon as he stopped eating his reactive foods, he was 75 percent improved. By dealing with his mold and pollen allergies, he was able to return to his former self.

While the "why" of chronic fatigue may be longer in coming, it's enough for the people like Christine, Denise, Trail, and Cleason, who have already found relief from their tiredness, to know that something as simple as removing their sensitive foods allowed them to return to normal lives.

CHAPTER 13

Migraine and Food Intolerance

"I used to have severe migraines two or three times a week," explains Sylvia. "During those attacks I became nauseous and tired. If I didn't have the chance to lie down, I had to take two or three very strong pain relievers to survive the day. On the weekends, I'd spend one or both days in bed. Now that I am no longer eating my intolerant foods, my migraines are completely gone. I'm so grateful to finally have relief and to live a normal life again."

This is one of many letters that thankful patients have written to Mr. Just Hintz, manager of a laboratory in Germany where doctors process their patients' ALCAT blood tests. And the writer is just one of many grateful migraine sufferers around the world who finally found relief—amid the various notions of how to treat migraines—after learning which foods their bodies tolerate, and by avoiding those foods. "We've found that most times, with migraines, patients improve," notes Hintz.

I've Got a Headache

Only a migraine sufferer can understand the excruciating, throbbing pain of this condition which, at its worse, can land a sufferer in bed for an occasional day or incapacitate them for several days each week. These debilitating headaches are often accompanied by vision sensitivities (even temporary blindness), nausea, shaking, vomiting, fatigue, depression, skin problems, and irritable bowel, all symptoms that compound the suffering. Statistically, each year in the U.S., headaches cripple more people than motorcycle accidents, car collisions, and industrial accidents combined. Over 45 million Americans get chronic, recurring headaches, and that number increases every year. Of this number, 16 to 18 million suffer from migraines, and 70 percent of all migraine sufferers are women.

These chronic, recurring headaches are severe enough to cause those in pain to seek medical attention and, in some cases, prevent them from maintaining full-time employment. According to the National Headache Foundation, by 1995 headaches cost industry a $50 billion loss due to absenteeism and medical expenses, and migraines caused sufferers to lose more than 157 million workdays. In excess of $4 billion is spent annually on over-the-counter pain relievers for headaches, many of which are ineffective.

In the United Kingdom, migraine sufferers comprise the largest group attending neurological clinics—up to one-third of all patients in some centers. Some estimates have placed the incidence of migraine in the population as high as 30 percent. In that country, more working days are lost due to headache than through any other single category of complaint. When migraineurs try to work with a headache, they are less efficient. And many feel they cannot plan their work and social lives for fear of being devastated by a headache.

Of the several types of headaches, most fall into one of three basic categories: tension-type headaches that bring an ache in the area where the muscles of the head and neck meet; vascular headaches, which include migraines, toxic, and cluster headaches; and organically caused headaches from tumors, infections, and disease. Many popular treatments are available—including prescription and over-the-counter medications, vertebra realignment, and psychotherapy—yet the excruciating head pain still continues for millions. Often sufferers search their whole lives for help, willing to try anything that even remotely claims to be a cure. Many choose to suffer the dangerous side effects of drugs, including constricted blood vessels around the heart as well as in the brain, rather than endure a migraine's wrath.

Some headache sufferers, however, have found the simple, drug-free solution—treatment for food intolerance. Thousands of patients and dozens of research studies show that identifying and eliminating their intolerant foods is a viable solution for many. How removing food (and chemical) intolerances works to alleviate migraines is not clear. Up to now, the cause of headaches has been attributed to hormonal imbalance, genetic predisposition, chronic tension, and emotional issues, with some foods cited as the triggers. However, physicians who recognize food intolerance as a cause of headaches agree that medical professionals who ignore food allergy cannot get the whole picture. As Dr. Richard Bahr, an environmental medicine specialist in Cincinnati, puts it: "We know that migraines are a food problem until you can prove otherwise. They are not all food-related, but the greater percent are."

"A large portion of head pain, including even the worst forms of migraine, are simply due to allergic reactions," writes Dr. Theron Randolph in *An Alternative*

Approach to Allergies. This simple fact has been the answer to many migraineurs' prayers. For example, Ruth, one of Dr. Ivonne Torre-Coya's migraine patients, found out through the ALCAT Test that she was intolerant to coffee and grapes, both of which she consumed frequently. "When she cut them out of her diet, the effect was incredible. Her headaches disappeared," explains Carmen, assistant to Dr. Torre-Coya, a physician and allergy specialist in Miami. "She was really happy, and feeling great."

Another grateful German patient who wrote to Mr. Hintz had this to say: "I took the ALCAT Test for my chronic sinus allergy problem, and after removing my allergenic foods, particularly wheat, there was a nice side effect—I don't have my migraines anymore, which I got quite often before."

Identifying "Trigger" Foods

It's common to hear that certain foods trigger migraines—for example, aged cheese, chocolate, and red wine are often implicated. But you'll never hear popular medical focus on lamb, milk, or wheat. Yet those are the foods that caused Tom, Sharon, and Barbara to suffer from excruciating headaches and migraines, no matter which of the commonly accepted headache-trigger foods they eliminated from their diets. Dr. Anthony Ferro in Palm Beach, who has successfully treated many patients with migraine, noted: "I have one patient, Tom, who gets a migraine whenever he eats wheat."

Sharon, a 52-year-old public relations consultant, is in generally good health except for severe migraines. For years she managed her migraines, which only occurred every once in awhile, by taking over-the-counter pain medications. Then, out of the blue, the migraines picked up in frequency and intensity; at least once a week she'd be way-laid by stabbing pain around the eyes and nausea that persisted for two hours. "I prefer not to take a lot of medications. But the increasingly severe headaches were starting to cut into my lifestyle. As a public relations consultant, I have a very active social life, and you don't exactly feel like going out dancing when you have a migraine."

Finally tested with the ALCAT Test at the suggestion of a business acquaintance, Sharon was surprised to learn that she was allergic to two of her favorite foods—lamb and chocolate—in addition to tomatoes, salmon, wheat, and dairy products, all of which she ate frequently. Looking back, she realized that her headaches had picked up in intensity when she started eating regularly at a new Mediterranean restaurant near her office. "I wasn't pleased to find out that I was reactive to foods I liked, so I decided to test the test. I ate lamb one day for lunch, and sure enough, an hour later I developed a migraine headache. I realized that there's a lot of validity here. With migraines, you don't want to test too much. But as per my doctor's recommendations, I did test it again a few months later and got another migraine within an hour or two of eating lamb. That was enough testing for me. Now I choose another dish at my favorite restaurant."

Dr. Barbara Solomon in Baltimore became interested in allergy in the mid-1960s when, as an internal medicine resident, she slowly started getting migraines. First she'd get one every three months, then monthly. Before long she was experiencing a migraine every week, then three times a week, until finally she had a constant migraine, including vomiting. This went on for a year until she could no longer stand the agonizing pain. Instinctively, she decided to try changing her diet. Since beef and milk were the main two foods in her busy life as a medical resident, she tried eliminating them. Dr. Solomon recalls:

I was amazed when the migraines went away. At the time, I didn't know about the research on food intolerance and headaches. But I thought: I'm not unique; there are other people with headaches and it's probably food related. If changing my diet worked for me, it might work for other people.

The first headache patient I tried this theory on ate nothing but cheese and wheat. So I advised him to cut both out of his diet, and I hit it right. When he didn't eat the foods, the headaches went away; when he ate them again, the headaches came back. I kept doing this with headache patients, and they kept getting better.

So every time I had a headache patient, I'd have them keep a food diary for a few weeks, then I'd advise them to give up the foods they ate the most frequently. Most of them got better. I'd challenge the result by having them add the foods back into their diets, and invariably they would get sick again. Then I decided that I had to have a test that could quickly tell me exactly to which foods my patients were intolerant. For nearly 20 years I used the only food intolerance testing method available at the time. But in the past 10 years I've been using the ALCAT Test. It's a much more convenient and efficient test.

Migraine and Intolerance:
Research Confirms the Connection

Dr. Solomon has since conducted research on the ALCAT Test to determine its effectiveness as a guide and barometer in the therapy of environmental and food sensitivities. Her study not only confirmed that the ALCAT Test is a valuable guide in quickly identifying a person's food, mold, and chemical allergies, but it also showed that several conditions, including migraines, can be improved by addressing food intolerance. "The traditional medical community says that classic migraine is not food allergy, but in my experience it is," says Dr. Solomon. Her study included 71 patients with headaches. Of the nine patients with classic migraine (which includes visual disturbances such as flashing lights and split vision), 82 percent showed improvement after eliminating the foods to which they tested reactive. Of the 39 patients with common migraine (which includes no visual disturbances), 62 percent showed improvement. And of the 23 patients with sinus headaches, 58 percent showed improvement. "My study showed that eliminating food intolerances is effective in clearing a person's migraine 82 percent of the time, and 82 percent is pretty good."

In two studies they conducted on migraines and food intolerance using the ALCAT Test, Drs. Fell and Brostoff found excellent results for headache and migraine sufferers. In the first study, conducted in 1988, 80 patients with a variety of conditions including migraine were observed. Drs. Fell and Brostoff showed that this simple blood test, as opposed to guesswork, enabled them to identify patients' food intolerance, and the patients who stopped eating the sensitive foods showed clear-cut improvement of migraines, while the patients who continued to eat their allergic foods showed "disastrous results." In a second study conducted in 1990, 14 of 18 patients with migraines got better. During the 12-month study, these patients' improvement was measured by scoring all four target symptoms—aura, headache, nausea, and vomiting. All maintained their success. "Interestingly, several of the patients said that although an aura developed, there was a failure of the full-blown syndrome to develop with headache, nausea, and vomiting," explains Brostoff.

A study on the relationship of food intolerance to weight loss, body composition, and self-reported disease symptoms was conducted in 1995 at the Columbia/HCA Medical Center's Sports Medicine and Performance Center in Houston and Baylor Medical College Sports Medicine and Performance Institute. Lead investigator Gilbert Kaats, Ph.D., director of the Health and Medical Research Foundation, an independent research organization in San Antonio, found that people on an ALCAT diet who reported suffering from migraines improved by 50 percent within four weeks. Migraine sufferers who followed diets of their own choosing said that their head pain had only improved by about 25 percent at the end of the four-week study.

The idea that allergenic foods can cause headaches is not new. Many researchers have discovered a relationship between allergy and migraines. As far back as 1905, the Australian medical pioneer Dr. Francis Hare reported that head pain could be the result of eating incompatible foods. In 1927, two prominent American allergists, Drs. Albert G. Rowe and Warren T. Vaughan, both published articles implicating specific foods as the cause of allergic headaches.

In a study in 1930, Dr. Rowe again found migraines to be related to food allergy. In 1934, Dr. A. Andresen reported that migraine was an allergic phenomenon. In 1979, Dr. C. G. Grant reported that diet led to freedom from migraine attacks in 51 of 60 patients, while the other nine patients experienced a reduction in headache frequency. In 1985, Dr. Lyndon Mansfield, president of the American In Vitro Allergy and Immunology Society and an allergy specialist in private practice in El Paso, Texas, published a study on food allergy and the adult migraine that showed a clear relationship between migraines and allergic disease. With guesswork alone to identify causative foods, Dr. Mansfield observed that 6 out of 43 patients became headache-free, and 13 subjects experienced 66 percent or greater reduction in headache frequency.

In 1935, Dr. Theron Randolph wrote a medical paper entitled "Allergy in Migraine-like Headaches," based on his work while at the University of Michigan Medical School. In this paper, he observed that two-thirds of the migraine patients at the University Hospital in Ann Arbor obtained relief from headaches by eliminating various foods from their diets. In 1989, he wrote, "These results are certainly better than those achieved by conventional medicine. There is no need for a person to suffer for years on end with persistent headaches when the cause of these disorders can often be identified and relieved by eliminating certain common substances from the environment. Today, however, even better results can be achieved through the diagnosis of chemical susceptibility and of some common food allergies, which had not then been identified." He notes that there is no mass-applicable shortcut to finding intolerant foods and controlling headaches. What affects one patient does not trouble the next. Individual testing using the ALCAT Test is needed.

Pain, Pain, Go Away: Children and Migraines

Adults are not the only ones to suffer from headaches and migraines; children do as well. Headaches in children are thought to be genetically inherited from parents who have migraines. Studies show that 70–80 percent of migraines have a hereditary influence. If both parents have them, children have a 75 percent chance of having migraines as well. When one parent suffers from migraines, the child will have a 50 percent chance of being afflicted. Dr. Joseph Egger, who works at the Chil-

drens' Hospital in Munich, Germany, posed the question
"Is Migraine Food Allergy?" in a study of children's headaches published in a 1983 issue of *The Lancet*. He found
that when 78 of 88 children who experienced headaches
at least once a week eliminated certain foods from their
diets, they completely recovered from the migraines, as
well as associated symptoms like abdominal pain, behavior disorders, asthma, and eczema.

---

*Many patients have been greatly
relieved to find a simple, noninvasive,
nonmedicating solution to their
children's debilitating headaches.*

This study also resulted in three interesting conclusions: (1) offending foods were most often unsuspected
and often the person's favorite foods; (2) although 17 of
the 88 subjects were allergic to only one food, the rest
were allergic to a number of foods; and (3) one child had
to eliminate 24 foods before getting relief from migraines.
Traditional allergy tests available at the time—skin tests
and RAST (radioallergosorbent test, a laboratory test specific for IgE antibodies)—were of no value in detecting
food intolerances.

Many parents have been greatly relieved to find a
simple, noninvasive, nonmedicating solution to their
children's debilitating headaches. At the suggestion of
Dr. John Gerrard, her children's physician and an expert

in allergy and immunology in Saskatchewan, Canada, Shirley removed sweets, chocolate, cola, and dairy products from her 12-year-old son Bruce's diet. His headaches went away.

Jackie's son Trent began having headaches and showing signs of hyperactivity at three years old. At the suggestion of her doctor, Jackie had Trent tested at age four using the ALCAT Test. While his hyperactivity rapidly improved by eliminating the intolerant foods, his migraines took a couple months to completely disappear. "I wasn't as concerned about the hyperactivity as I was about the migraines," explains Jackie. "They were frightening when he got then. He'd have no motor skills for nearly two hours. I don't like to give my child medications. And although it's not easy to feed a young child food they like, if I can alter his diet that is definitely the lesser of two evils." Consistent with the research on the hereditary nature of migraines, Jackie says that she herself had developed migraines while she was pregnant.

Lorraine says that when her children's fifth doctor, Dr. Constantine Kotsanis, a pediatrician in Dallas, suggested food and chemical allergies as an answer to her six-year-old son's attention-deficit-hyperactivity disorder, her four-year-old daughter's autism, and both children's accompanying headaches, she "didn't know what to think. No doctor had ever said anything about allergy being the problem before." Dr. Kotsanis has successfully treated many children with ADHD and other conditions by uncovering their food intolerances using the ALCAT Test. Lorraine's daughter had to eliminate corn, tomato, tuna, shrimp, and blue dye, and avoid some specific molds. Her son had to eliminate chicken, sugar, broccoli, sulfites, and red dye, and avoid most molds.

Like many children, Lorraine's kids responded well to dietary changes. "I was so relieved to find a solution to the migraines. My daughter's were so painful she would bang herself on the head. It seemed like she was always in pain, and it was running me ragged. Now, she no longer bangs herself on the head and her grouchiness and stomachaches are gone. What's more, she is much more receptive to learning than ever before. But if she eats corn or tomatoes, she'll start flying around the room. My six-year-old son had always complained about tummy-ache and headache after eating and now his pain is gone." She says by changing her children's diets, her headaches have gone away, too.

Virginia wishes that doctors had diagnosed her food intolerances when she was a child. If they had, it would have saved her years of pain. As a child Virginia loved cookies and candy as much as the next child and she ate them as often as she could. But she had something her playmates didn't have—severe headaches. Her parents took her to several doctors, "none of whom ever mentioned food allergy being a possible cause to my headaches," Virginia says. Finally, in her teen and college years, her headaches disappeared and she thought she was free from the excruciating pain. Then as a teacher and young mother raising three children, the headaches came back with a vengeance as full-blown migraines, landing her in bed, heavily medicated, at least once a week.

Virginia went to Dr. Anthony Ferro in West Chester, Pennsylvania, for her headaches after the doctor had successfully cured her son's sinus problem. Dr. Ferro ran an ALCAT Test and found her intolerant to several foods, including chocolate, yeast, sugar, eggplant, and green peppers. "Chocolate is totally out," she says. "It gives me such a bad headache, I can't ever eat it. I don't indulge in yeast and sugar much at all. I can have a little bit of green pepper, eggplant, and other nightshade vegetables, but if I ate them every day I'd be in bad shape. Looking back, I realize that during the time I was headache-free, in my teens and during college, was a period when I didn't eat desserts very often."

Virginia went on a bland diet, including completely eliminating her intolerant foods, for six months at the beginning of her therapy to rid her body of the antibiotics she'd been taking to fight her annual bouts of strep throat. While on the bland diet she didn't have a single headache. Since she's been off the bland diet, she has had a few headaches, but nothing like before. She attributes her current headaches to the fact that she is not especially strict with her diet:

"If I do eat desert, I try to eat one with less sugar. I can't even overdo on honey and fruit. I can only have one piece of bread a day because of yeast. I feel really healthy these days. I've only had one bad cold that required antibiotics. I am really grateful to find a solution to controlling the pain, lethargy, and irritability, because the migraines were becoming a definite problem." Like a lot of patients who eliminated foods for symptoms unrelated to weight, Virginia also lost an extra ten pounds she'd been carrying.

The Anatomy of a Migraine

The physical process and cause of headaches and migraines are not yet clearly understood. Current thinking suggests that the aura, or warning associated with migraine (such as vision problems), is due to a narrowing or constriction of the blood vessels supplying the brain and its surrounding tissues, thereby reducing the blood flow to the areas. Following the constriction phase, the blood vessels are then believed to dilate more than normal. The typical pounding headache and migraine is associated with the swelling of the blood vessels surrounding the brain.

Another part of this stage is inflammation caused by the clumping of certain blood cells, the platelets, during an attack. These platelets are tiny cell-type structures in the blood whose main function is to help the blood clot around a wound. During clotting the platelets clump together and release the natural brain neurotransmitter serotonin, which makes the blood vessels constrict to help reduce blood loss. During a migraine attack, the platelets clump together and release large amounts of serotonin when it is not needed. The serotonin makes the blood vessels constrict and so reduces the blood flow to the brain.

The body has control mechanisms that counteract the effect of the serotonin, but these may cause a violent swing in the opposite direction when they come into play. Interestingly, the eicosanoids PGE-2 and PGI-1 are both potent vasodilators. PGE-2 is found in areas of inflammation and is synthesized by platelets, while PGI-1 is synthesized by the blood vessel lining or endothelium and is an antagonist of platelet clumping. The increased production of these eicosanoids in response to the inflammation and platelet clumping associated with a food sensitivity reaction may partially explain many migraine headache reactions. The blood vessels in the brain open up too much, which brings on the throbbing pain that is a feature of the second phase of the attack. At this point increased pressure on certain parts of the brain might produce feelings of nausea.

The ALCAT Test measures the change in the size and number of white blood cells and also identifies when foods or chemicals cause platelet clumping. (This serotonin-induced constriction of the vasculature may explain how fenfluramine [of "phen-fen" fame] and its related compound, dexfenfluramine [trade name Redux] lead to an increased risk for primary pulmonary hypertension [PPH] and associated heart valve damage.)

Flawed Theories

Two popular theories regarding how severe headaches and migraines come about relate to specific food "triggers" and hormonal changes. Yet eliminating foods such as chocolate, aged cheese, and red wine and taking hormone-managing drugs such as nonsteroidal, anti-inflammatory agents have helped few sufferers. The "amines" in certain foods are thought to affect the diameter of the blood vessels, and thereby produce headaches. (Amines are byproducts of chemical reactions involving amino acids in the body, but also exist naturally in certain foods. The most common reference is to foods high in tyramine. Tyramine is neutralized in the bodies of most people by monamine oxidase.)

But research has shown that "there must be other factors that can make the platelets clump together, because it is only a minority of patients whose migraines are triggered by these foods," says Dr. Brostoff. He continues by describing the process:

> The foods identified by an elimination diet seem to be acting in a different way from the accepted food "triggers." When these foods are eliminated from the diet, the migraines usually clear up completely, whereas excluding trigger foods only makes the migraines less frequent. Following an elimination diet, and the avoidance of culprit foods, patients often find that they can once more tolerate their triggers—both food and nonfood. It looks as if the milk, wheat, or whatever was creating some serious underlying problem that made the body vulnerable to any external change.
>
> Thus bright lights, stress, the flickering of a television screen, or the pharmacologically active substances in chocolate could upset the delicate balance and tip the whole system into a migraine attack. Once the underlying food intolerance has been sorted out, the system is far more stable

and can better cope with external circumstances. . . . One of the main preventive measures is to minimize the "load" by excluding the worst offenders or minimizing the lesser offenders. There is a threshold beyond which a migraine attack is triggered; to lower the load so that the threshold is never reached enables the individual to maintain health rather than to have to treat an illness.

Eliminating our system's reactive foods is the fastest, most effective way to reduce the "load" on our system.

Hormonal changes have also been implicated as a cause of migraines due to the fact that migraines affect women more than men, and they often begin occurring at the onset of menstruation. However, if female endocrine changes are to blame, the current treatment of choice—drugs—is a poor solution for most people. According to an article in the January/February 1996 issue of *Health* magazine, written by Dr. Fred Sheftell, director and co-founder of the New England Center for Headache, the migraine pharmaceuticals don't work for everyone, and can have dangerous side effects. Interestingly, the drugs mimic the neurotransmitter serotonin by constricting blood vessels. However, the drugs show no discretion in which blood vessels they constrict; along with brain blood vessels, they constrict blood vessels leading to the heart, legs, and arms—which can lead to potentially severe health problems.

"If you're born with this disorder, it's like having a stick of dynamite with a fuse in your head, and certain activators—stress, foods, hormonal fluctuations—light it," Dr. Sheftell says. The article further reported that migraine sufferers are waiting for the "breakthrough drug" or the "perfect fix" that will block migraines by reducing the inflammation in their head without affecting arteries or veins in other parts of the body. They just don't know yet that thousands of migraine sufferers have *already* discovered the perfect fix—eliminating intolerant foods. What could be safer or more natural than that?

Further, patients are rarely aware of the environmental source of their illness. You may see no relation between eating and your headaches, since the effects can be delayed (from one hour to seven days). Or you may know that your headache is somehow related to food intake, but that intake is so complex and varied that uncovering the actual source may seem impossible. Or you may know that a particular food *relieves* your headache pain, not realizing that the "relief" meal is nothing but your maintenance dose.

Serotonin is a chemical substance primarily present in the platelets. This neurotransmitter, which is also naturally produced in the brain, has the job of sending messages between nerve cells, thereby controlling how we feel. Serotonin may have different effects when it is produced in the brain to serve as a neurotransmitter as opposed to being released into the bloodstream as a result of an inflammatory reaction and platelet clumping. Vasodilatation may be viewed as the body's tendency to return to normal following the vasoconstriction associated with a food reaction and platelet clumping.

As Dr. Solomon puts it: "With any condition, unless you remove all the foods that trigger a person's migraines, you're not going to get to the problem."

CHAPTER 14

Food Intolerance: How to Live with It

Once you know or suspect food intolerance, the treatment is avoiding offending food. In our fast-food, multiethnic food-oriented society, this can be quite a challenge. Treatment of food intolerance requires commitment and focus. For the most part, you will need to prepare foods at home to be sure reactive foods are carefully excluded. This can be an imposition if you eat most meals out. That doesn't change the fact that you must eliminate your offending foods before your symptoms will subside.

Eat Safely

The most practical approach to eliminating reactive foods is to assimilate a list of "safe" foods. Such a list is provided along with ALCAT Test results. Your ALCAT list of foods is divided into four parts, each containing representative foods from each major food family to be eaten on four consecutive days. This helps you plan meals in which no food is repeated more frequently than every four days, yet ensures that you'll get the needed vitamins and minerals to maintain good nutrient health. By using the "safe" foods in this way, you minimize intolerance to new foods and achieve variety and diversity by exploring new food choices rather than coveting your old favorites.

While following your elimination diet, you'll find it best to stick to simple basic meals and avoid complicated recipes and dishes, which concentrate too many food choices in a single meal and often severely limit later meal choices. After about two weeks, you might anticipate improvement of any symptoms associated with food intolerance. Any symptoms associated with reactive foods will continue to subside if you continue to avoid foods to which you are sensitive.

Become a Detective

If some symptoms linger, you may need to further eliminate suspicious foods, probably those that are a regular part of your diet. You might, for example, eliminate wheat, corn, milk, peanuts, tomatoes, and soy if you haven't already eliminated them. While others may well be the real culprits, the ones mentioned are so insidious in American processed foods that they easily slip into elimination diets. Strategically eliminating these foods in conjunction with your known reactive foods may lead to relief of your symptoms. At this point, you might contact a professional acquainted with strict elimination diets to help you seek out the culprit food.

A curious and as yet unexplained phenomenon of food sensitivity is that you may need to eliminate all your reactive foods before your symptoms will subside since they may represent reactions to food combinations rather than to individual foods. For that reason, eliminating individual reactive foods one at a time and using relief of symptoms as your endpoint is not a reliable method.

Should you test positive to a large number of foods, rather than assume the imposing task of eliminating this mass of favorite foods in one swift stroke, choosing five or six foods to eliminate the first week is less painful. Then you can add more foods to your elimination list for the second week and so on until you have included all your reactive foods. This method allows you to adapt to your new diet without the shock of losing all your standby foods at once. Nonetheless, you must eliminate all your reactive foods at the same time to expect the best results.

Identify Your Reactive Foods

You'll find the ALCAT Test results in an informative guide to your reactive foods. You will find a complete list of all the foods tested in the front of the guide. Each food will be accompanied by a rating of either "negative," "1+", "2+," or "MPOS."

The "negative" foods are those to which you demonstrate no allergic reaction. These represent your "safe" foods and should be the foundation of your diet plan as you eliminate your reactive foods.

The "1+" foods are those to which you exhibited a reaction, but of an equivocal nature. That is to say, only a small percentage of the white blood cells and/or platelets showed signs of response. These foods may represent potential intolerance, but for the most part should be consumed cautiously. Eating these foods no more often than once a week will allow you to determine whether or not they contribute to your symptoms. If you had very few foods in the "2+" or "MPOS" range, you should eliminate those in the "1+" range. Reactive foods may fall into the "1+" range erroneously if you were taking certain anti-inflammatory medications, antihistamines, or steroids when the test was administered.

If you are not losing weight by exercising regularly and are hungry after exercising, consider testing for food sensitivities.

Foods in the "2+" range are those to which you are likely to be intolerant. Curiously, you may find some foods in this category that you rarely or never eat. Because this may represent genetically determined intolerance, you are wise to continue to avoid these foods. Foods in the "2+" range represent foods to which your cells exhibited significant signs of reaction. You should eliminate these foods from your diet meticulously for a period of at least three months, after which you may reintroduce them into your diet to evaluate its intolerance. Food intolerance is different from allergic reactions in that the body may cease to react to the food after a period of elimination. When reintroducing foods, add only one food at a time. Eat normal quantities of this food on a single day, then wait three days before you reintroduce any others. If no characteristic symptoms develop, you may incorporate the food into your four-day rotation diet plan.

Foods in the "MPOS" range represent those foods that elicited the maximum positive reaction from your body's cells. These foods, like those in the "2+" range, should be strictly eliminated for a period of at least three months before you attempt to reintroduce them. Keep in mind that the degree of reactivity does not accurately establish the cause of symptoms. Symptoms may result from any of your reactive foods. The degrees of reaction only represent the intensity with which your blood cells reacted to a particular food in the test.

In many cases, individual reactive foods may cause symptoms only when they are eaten along with other reactive foods; the combination of these foods may cause you problems. Strictly avoiding all your reactive foods is the most practical way to eliminate food allergy symptoms.

Avoid Your Intolerant Foods

Following the report of your degree of reactivity to various foods is a concise listing of your reactive foods and their close relatives. This is a useful list to copy and keep in the car, purse or briefcase, and kitchen. Having this list available at strategic times when you are shopping or preparing food will lessen the likelihood of inadvertently eating foods you should eliminate.

You will notice that class 1+ reactive foods do not appear on this list unless you had very few 2+ or MPOS foods. You should consider class 1+ reactive foods "equivocal" unless they are the predominant reactive category. If class 1+ foods appear here, you should eliminate them completely since they may represent the maximum reaction the body is able to muster under certain conditions. Also, keep in mind that using anti-inflammatory medication, steroids, and antihistamines may alter the body's reaction to an allergen.

Stick to Your Eating List

This list of "safe" foods that should make up the foundation of your diet plan is your gold mine. Foods to which you tested negative are unlikely to be reactive for you. Take some time to carefully review this list. Most represent staples you are familiar with or reasonable substitutes you may never have tried because the local grocery didn't find them profitable. It is important to begin to realize how much we are at the mercy of the retailer's bottom line when we shop for food.

Don't be put off by the sometimes unusual names. Most foods on this list can be found at progressive grocers or at health-food stores. You will soon appreciate this if you are intolerant of common foods such as corn, wheat, milk, eggs, or soy. Our packaged food industry makes prolific use of common foods—in fact, about 75 percent of the foods in a package at a grocery contain corn or corn products. No wonder corn shows up on the list of ten foods to which people are most likely to be intolerant. Use this information to realize how important it is to vary your foods from day to day.

Follow a Four-Day Rotation Diet

This section conveniently separates all your "safe" foods into four consecutive days to ensure you will not eat any one food more than once in the four-day cycle. It is a useful way to juggle the large list of foods you may eat. There is nothing sacred about the particular arrangement of these foods, and you may switch foods to different days if you wish. The important thing to remember is that once you switch a food, you should eat it no more often than every fourth day to minimize the prospect of developing new food intolerance while on your elimination diet.

General Information

What follows in the manual is a computer-generated information section to assist you in planning your meals. Understand that this section does not take into account your individual food intolerance. You should read this section only to reinforce your dietary planning—not to justify eating a food to which you are reactive.

Your Reactive Food Information

I consider this section the most informative in the manual. Here you will learn more about your reactive foods and how to avoid them, than you will ever need to know. Full of insights to avoid ruining your elimination diet plan, this section bears careful attention.

Treating Candida Albicans

This particular reactive test is worth discussing separately. If you tested positive to *candida,* you will have noticed that the list of foods you are allowed is exceptionally small. This is because all sugars, starches, and yeast-containing foods have been eliminated.

Candida survives in your intestine by living on simple carbohydrates. Eliminating this food supply is necessary to kill the yeast. Testing positive to candida means that your immune system detected the organism in your bloodstream at some time. Candida can spread via the bloodstream to other organs and become a serious life-threatening problem in cases of a severely compromised immune system (such as during chemotherapy or in persons with cancer). The fact that candida was detected in your bloodstream at all justifies aggressive dietary treatment. Many physicians prefer aggressive drug treatment of candida at the time of dietary restriction, so you may want to consult with your physician regarding this. An excellent resource for those testing positive to candida is *The Yeast Connection* by William Crook, M.D.

Taking the Challenge Test

The challenge test is a mechanism for testing previously eliminated foods to evaluate their reactivity (or tendency to cause symptoms). This is accomplished by meticulously eliminating a food for a period of greater than two weeks, by which time your body will react differently if you are truly reactive to the food. When you reintroduce the food after two weeks of elimination, the typical reaction may be of a hyper-reactive nature—more immediate and more intense than previously noticed. For this reason it is best to challenge only test foods that were equivocal in their allerginicity (1+). Paying careful attention to your symptoms for the next three days should establish the safety index of the food. If a food does not elicit reactions when challenge tested, you may include it in your four-day elimination diet plan. However, if challenge testing a food results in return of your symptoms, strictly eliminate the food from the diet for a period of three to six months before you repeat challenge testing. If a food persists in precipitating symptoms after three months, you should eliminate it for one year before retesting.

The good news is that much food intolerance resolves after three months of strict elimination. The exact mechanism for this is not known. Remember that people with food intolerance tend toward food intolerance in the future. The practice of rotating foods on a four-day schedule is useful in decreasing the likelihood of your food intolerances reoccurring.

The above descriptions of food elimination and challenge testing are particularly applicable if you present the overt physical symptoms often associated with food intolerance. If your primary symptom of food intolerance is overweight, you must take a different approach.

In case of food intolerance as a cause of overweight, the culprit foods should be eliminated for three months. Then they should be reintroduced only on a four-day rotating basis. Challenge testing is not beneficial if the only physical evidence of intolerance is overweight. It is relatively easy to notice the sudden onset of sinus congestion, headache, or fatigue, but quite another to evaluate a subtle change in weight when you are challenge-testing a food.

Talk will not conquer obesity as a public health menace. Drugs have not decreased deaths from obesity. It is time for the individual to guide his or her health care and destiny relating to weight. Take a proactive position regarding your health by learning how to identify and eliminate your reactive foods. Congratulations on your major commitment to protect your health through the elimination of your reactive foods.

"Let Thy Food Be Thy Medicine"

No single aspect of American life influences our health more than does the food we eat. As we finally set out to eliminate overweight and its incredible burden on society, our focus must be on the food we eat and its relationship to the diseases that kill us prematurely. Our food makes many of us fat because we react inappropriately to it.

According to the March 9, 1998, *PRNewswire,* James M. Rippe, M.D., of the Center for Clinical and Lifestyle Research and Tufts University School of Medicine, urges physicians to treat obesity as an independent health problem rather than simply treating its common consequences—such as coronary heart disease, hypertension,

Type II diabetes, and elevated blood lipids. Dr. Rippe emphasized that while data clearly support the positive effects of weight loss on reducing health risk, physicians have not taken an active role in treating obesity. He also states: "Traditionally, physicians have failed to treat obesity in their patients. . . . Identifying patients early and starting long-term obesity treatment including diet, exercise and new pharmacotherapies when appropriate can save lives. We must attack obesity to attack the root of the problem."

As this book establishes, unrecognized and untreated food intolerance is a cause of overweight, as well as a cause of migraine headaches, sinus congestion, attention-deficit disorder, arthritis, fatigue, irritable bowel syndrome, colitis, gastritis, skin rashes, and depression. Yet as we search for an explanation of overweight, it will almost certainly be outside the traditional concepts of conventional medical philosophy. Years of research and study have failed to explain why people lose and regain unwanted weight except to note people gain weight when they eat too much.

But we can now keep the wild animal inside of us at bay. Without spending weeks trying and trading foods to determine which may be causing our problems, we can put information in front of us by taking the ALCAT Test. By avoiding the reactive foods the test identifies, we reopen doors long since shut in our face. Again in control, we can watch our weight melt away as our cravings disappear and food no longer holds our mind hostage. Clean out the cupboards, review basic nutrition, and cull bad habits; it's a whole new lifestyle. So redeeming is the freedom from the limitations of food intolerance that the words from the old spiritual quoted by Reverend Martin Luther King come to mind: "Free at last, free at last, thank God Almighty, free at last."

Food elimination as a cure for disease, often referred to as "alternative medicine," now takes the spotlight by default. Nothing else has worked. Again we appreciate the value of the earliest medical advice given 2,500 years ago by Hippocrates, the father of medicine: "Let thy food be thy medicine and thy medicine be thy food." The science and art of eliminating or prescribing food for the relief of illness has always been medicinal. Conventional intervention might better be considered "alternative medicine." Identifying and eliminating intolerant foods is the new "medicine" to conquer obesity.

Frequently Asked Questions
about Food Sensitivities

Food intolerance represents a new and radical reform in health care that conflicts with many conventional concepts of food and eating. These conventional approaches have perpetuated overweight and confused the general population. Following are answers to some of the commonly asked questions regarding the cause and treatment of overweight.

Q Doctor, I exercise regularly and try to eat healthy, but I can't seem to lose weight. Could food sensitivities be part of my problem?

A Yes, food intolerance may well be a part of your problem in losing weight. Normally when we exercise we tap into our fat stores for energy. Aerobic exercise is the best form of exercise to consume fat because fat must be oxidized to utilize it as energy. Therefore exercise classified as aerobic (that is, "with air") would be the best choice of exercise if one's goal were to decrease body fat stores. In the case of food-intolerant individuals, the chemical reaction of the allergic food seems to prevent the efficient use of fat for energy.

The exact mechanism of this has yet to be determined, but if you tend to become increasingly hungry after exercise, your body is telling you that your exercise was financed with your emergency energy stores of glycogen, emergency energy stores found in your liver and muscle. Once you have tapped these emergency stores, your body will insist that you replenish this energy as soon as possible to be ready for the next emergency. Needless to say, this is not the ideal energy source for someone trying to lose fat weight by exercising. In fact, a number of patients gained fat as well as muscle weight when they began exercise programs. This was a result of their increased hunger after exercise, which they tended to satisfy with carbohydrate and fat snacks. The end result was that the fat was stored and became part of the problem they were trying to eliminate.

Fortunately, once they eliminated foods to which they were intolerant, they began to notice more appropriate changes in their body composition (lean tissue to fat ratio) in response to regular aerobic exercise. As an added bonus, they were not hungry after exercise because they did not have to replenish their emergency energy stores. Exercise should alleviate hunger, not make it worse. If you are not losing fat weight by exercising regularly and are hungry after exercising, consider testing for food sensitivities.

Q **Using medication I can consistently lose weight for a couple of months but as soon as I stop the medication I start gaining it back. Should I just stay on the medicine permanently?**

A If anyone requires medication permanently, their doctor has apparently exhausted all other means to diagnose and treat their condition. As far as I know, no one who is overweight suffers from low blood levels of appetite suppressants any more than headache is caused by aspirin deficiency. So, taking them on a permanent basis is probably not the best solution to the problem. Before you give up, be sure that you and your doctor are delving into all the possible causes of your overweight. These may include candidiasis, thyroid disorders, pituitary disorders, genetically inherited disorders, poor eating habits, nutritional deficiencies, emotional eating, stress eating, and obviously food intolerance. (The list is actually longer but you get the idea.) The odds are that with nutritional guidance and real lifestyle changes, you can probably deal with the problem of overweight without the crutch of appetite suppressants. Find a doctor who is interested in eliminating all the likely underlying causes of your overweight.

Q **I can't seem to lose weight after my doctor stopped giving me Pondomin and recently found a source of Pondomin from Mexico. Would it be okay for me to take it from time to time?**

A No. There is no good reason to risk your health taking a drug that has been taken off the market in America. Our health-care system may have many faults, but ignoring evidence that a drug may be dangerous to use would be foolish and irresponsible.

　　Find a doctor who will help you discover the underlying cause of your overweight and treat it appropriately. The quick fix is always a bad idea. The lifestyle we live in America is so fast paced that we often don't spend time taking care of ourselves. The price we pay is a lifetime of frustration with frequent quick trips to the doctor. Until we become responsible for our actions and treat our bodies with respect, medicine is not going to be the answer. Real treatment of any disease involves the partnership of your doctor's knowledge and your commitment to become healthy.

Q **Doctor, I have severe adult acne, terrible migraine headaches, and am about 75 pounds overweight. No one has been able to help me with these problems. How come our medical system that can transplant hearts can't do more for my problems?**

A To dissect the politics and economics of medicine in this country is beyond the scope of this response. Suffice it to say that your doctors haven't yet found the underlying cause of your problems. Although all of your conditions may be related to food sensitivities, there certainly are a variety of other possible etiologies. Nonetheless, if you haven't been tested for food sensitivities, it would be worthwhile to do so. Many people find that eliminating reactive foods gives them long overdue relief from chronic conditions thought to be incurable.

Q **Doctor, how can you be so sure that food sensitivities are the cause of overweight?**

A I can't be sure that food sensitivities are the cause of everyone's overweight. Overweight has become a national stigma and its "cause" has evaded definition to date. I do know that weight loss evaded many of my patients until they eliminated foods identified by sensitivity testing. We all know that eating too much food will lead to over-weight. What we may be overlooking is that in some cases "too much" may be only a bite of the wrong food. Food intolerance as a cause of overweight makes remarkable good sense—as the "cause of the cause" of overweight. That is, food intolerance results in overeating of foods which, while they increase serotonin levels, also increase fat deposits. That answer was a bit more complicated than I like, but I'm sure you get the idea.

Q **Doctor, do you think I can lose weight if I find out what foods I am sensitive to?**

A I am pretty sure you will *not* lose weight if you *only* find out to which foods you are sensitive. To benefit from knowl-edge of food intolerance, you must eliminate the culprit foods, and this means *ELIMINATE* in most cases. If you are unable to completely eliminate the culprit foods for the necessary period of time, allowing your body to "for-get" the sensitivity, you may well suffer relapses. This can be avoided by seeking the help of a professional who can advise you as to "challenge testing" (introducing foods one at a time to see whether you still react adversely to a food) as well as healthy nutritional balance to prevent the likelihood of acquiring new food intolerance.

Q Doctor, I know my reactive foods, but my weight loss seems slow, only a pound or two each week. Is there anything I can do to speed this up?

A First of all, my calculations show that at a pound or two each week, you would lose between 50 and 100 pounds a year, which is plenty of weight to lose in a year. The need for immediate gratification is a fault we are all guilty of from time to time. Practical healthy physiologic limits to weight loss permit all the involved body systems to synchronize their functions as the burden of overweight is removed.

Rather than fixating on weight loss per se, you would do well to sit down with a health professional you respect and identify your eating triggers—emotional eating, stress eating, pleasure eating, for example. Make a plan for healthy lifestyle changes that will maintain your successful weight loss. Implementing these changes gradually as you lose weight will give you the confidence needed to keep the weight off. It is important to discover and resolve all the precipitating forces involved in overeating to prevent relapse.

Q Doctor, I am having trouble finding foods that taste good to me on my elimination diet; I am attracted to my familiar foods. Is it okay for me to mix some of my reactive foods with my "safe" foods to give them some taste?

A Nice try, but sorry, you must eliminate your reactive foods to prevent the allergic reaction in your body. Sneaking or "accidentally on purpose" eating your reactive foods will result in having to start over the necessary elimination period. Curiously, you may find that you experience a hyperacute reaction to these foods if you eat them before your body has completely given them the seal of approval. This means you may experience an intense, rapid reaction after eating the food that had been incompletely eliminated. From my experience, such a reaction is great incentive to stick to your elimination diet.

If you eliminate saturated fats and all sweets during your elimination time frame, you will find that natural foods taste different and better than you remembered. It seems that fats and sugar are so stimulating to the taste buds that nothing else can quite compare. This leads us to search for more fats and sugar to equal the taste "intoxication" mode of eating. How often have you heard someone rave so about a fatty, sugary treat that you would think it was as healthy as mother's milk? They are eating for taste to the exclusion of nutrition.

Q If I can never eat these foods again, what will I do if I develop intolerance to the foods I am allowed?

A Good question. First of all, remember that for some reason not completely understood, the immune system often "forgets" a delayed food allergy if it doesn't come in contact with the food for a period of time. This may represent an eccentricity of the immune system that allowed early man to feast on foods in season. When not available, man essentially eliminated them from his diet and never suffered the long-term effects of food intolerance. In modern times, we must work at eliminating foods from the diet because they are available year-round. It is generally recognized that after a period of three to six months, reactive foods may be reintroduced into the diet. To decide whether a food remains reactive, it is reintroduced in normal amounts and observed for renewal of symptoms for a period of three days. It is important to "challenge" test only one food at a time. An alternative would be to repeat the ALCAT Test every three to six months.

Secondly, it is important to avoid the development of new food intolerance while on your elimination diet. This is accomplished by eating slowly, varying your foods through rotation diet planning, enhancing immune system nutrition through diet and supplements, and doing something to alleviate the stress in your life.

Q **I have lost weight using a commercial weight-loss program, but regained the weight soon after leaving the program. How would food intolerance explain this?**

A Most commercial weight-loss programs focus on calorie reduction and exercise to effect weight loss. Until the underlying causes of overweight are identified and treated, the condition is likely to recur. Food intolerance may play a role in these programs in that the diets and supplements prescribed are a "one-size-fits-all" program. That is, their profit is to be made from sales of food and food supplements and exchanges designed to lower caloric intake overall. This is without regard for food intolerance. If an individual is intolerant of a food or a food component of the supplement, weight loss and maintenance is going to be unlikely. Likewise if the individual eliminates his reactive food for only a short period of time, the allergic reaction will likely resume as he or she resumes their "regular" diet.

Any weight-loss program can be enhanced through the use of the ALCAT Test to identify reactive foods. You should eliminate these foods in addition to the other modalities to effectively lose and keep weight off.

Q **Why do I crave some of the foods I am sensitive to?**

A This curious aspect of food intolerance is not yet well understood, though some suggest it may represent withdrawal. When the chemical reactions precipitated by the allergic response are pleasurable, the absence of this allergic response results in unpleasant feelings, which can only be remedied by eating the food and creating the allergic reaction again.

Another interesting theory compares food sensitivities to serum sickness. The body produces excessive antibodies to a food such that the individual is actually sick from their own antibodies. Only when the food antigen is reintroduced and binds with the antibodies does the condition improve. Unfortunately the food stimulates more antibodies and the cycle repeats.

More research is needed to define this aspect of food sensitivities. Until the answers are in, your best efforts should be directed toward eliminating your reactive foods.

Q My two brothers and my mother are allergic to wheat. Am I likely to be allergic to wheat also?

A Maybe. Evidence suggests that some food intolerance may be genetically programmed. Although each individual is different, certain tendencies are genetically predetermined. For example, if one's ancestors never developed the enzyme systems to metabolize milk byproducts, the body may protect itself from toxic overload through allergic response to discourage drinking of milk in all its descendants. Interesting observations in Denmark have revealed similar sensitivities in identical twins. Although this is interesting, thorough testing is still necessary to determine one's food sensitivities. Further study is necessary to establish any useful predictive value to one family member's food intolerance.

Q How I can be sensitive to a food I have never eaten?

A This question comes up frequently as we review test results with patients. The answer again lies in genetic predisposition. People may be genetically programmed to be intolerant of a food. This may occur without their ever having been exposed to the food. The good news is that if one has never been exposed to the food, it is obviously not a favorite food and therefore not a problem to eliminate. Genetically modulated food intolerances are, however, of a more permanent nature than immune system modulated intolerances. If you find you are intolerant of a food you don't ever remember eating, you will probably always have a reaction to that food. So, it would be best to continue not eating it. Be aware, however, that the food in question may be present in some prepared foods without your realizing it.

Q **My seasonal pollen allergies have improved tremendously since I have eliminated my reactive foods. Can food allergies make pollen allergies worse?**

A Many patients realize an improvement in symptoms of airborne allergies after eliminating reactive foods. In some cases the mechanism may be one of cross-reactivity. We know, for example, that sensitivity to apples is predictive of sensitivity to Birch pollen, and sensitivity to cantaloupe is often coupled with sensitivity to ragweed. Once the food sensitivity is resolved, the airborne allergy may also improve or disappear.

Another interesting aspect of food intolerance is the relationship of co-factors. You may not typically react to a food but may react to the same food if you eat it following exercise. Or you may only react to a food seasonally when certain pollen co-factors are present. Often another food is the inciting co-factor, without which there is no apparent reaction. This aspect of food intolerance is a "gray area" but symptomatically responds well to removal of either of the co-factor components.

Q **My elimination diet leaves me very little food that I care to eat. Would I be able to use the protein drinks at the health-food stores as meal substitutes until I can re-introduce some of my foods?**

A I would encourage you to explore the many foods listed as the foods you may eat. Although these may seem strange to you, I believe you will find them not unlike their common cousins, to which you are more accustomed. Expanding your food choices is a benefit in terms of nutrition.

Commercially prepared protein meal substitutes are generally not a good idea on your elimination diet. These commercial concoctions are more often than not made from a wide variety of substances known to be allergenic. The protein in these meal replacements is usually derived from egg, soy, and milk protein, all of which are high on the list of common reactive substances. To make matters worse, many of these formulas contain large amounts of hidden sugars and chemicals to improve the taste.

If a packaged meal substitute were needed for traveling or just to avoid the inconvenience of preparing food during the day, the ATML Corp. has available a hypoallergenic protein formula. This proprietary formula is a rich and healthy protein base, chemical-free and vitamin-enriched, which is more appropriate for the food-intolerant individual. Taste-wise it is better than most protein meal substitutes and is appropriate for anyone not intolerant of rice.

Fast track to staying well   If you get sick, assume it was something you ate that you shouldn't have or something you didn't eat that you should have; and don't do it again.

BIBLIOGRAPHY OF SELECTED ALCAT TEST STUDIES

The studies below are a sampling of international ALCAT Test studies and results that confirm the effectiveness of the Test.

Cabo-Soler, J. Comments on diets in esthetic medicine. Presented at the 14th Mediterranean Day of Esthetical Medicine and Dermatological Surgery, Venice, Italy, Sept. 22–23, 1995.

This Spanish study was designed to determine whether people who could not lose weight on a low calorie diet could resume their weight loss using the results from the ALCAT Test

Using a group of 30 patients who had difficulty losing weight when they adhered to a reduced calorie diet, this study confirmed a greater weight loss in almost all the patients when they were placed on a diet planned according to the ALCAT Test results. Also, the weight loss was mostly fat, with minor muscle loss. In some cases, muscle mass was increased.

Other interesting observations included (1) improved skin smoothness, (2) a loss of fat from the thigh area, making it useful in planning a diet to control cellulitis, (3) a better sense of well being and improved physical performance, and (4) improvement in abdominal bloating and digestive problems.

These findings are significant because many overweight patients find it difficult to lose weight by cutting calories alone. This study suggests that delayed food allergies may interfere with weight loss regardless of calorie restriction. Also, the beneficial effects of skin smoothness, loss of fat from the thigh area, improved sense of well being, and improvement of gastrointestinal conditions were bonuses to those following the ALCAT diet plan

Fell B., J. Brostoff, and M. Pasula. "High Correlation of the ALCAT Test Results with Double-Blind Challenge in Food Sensitivity." Paper presented at the 45th annual Congress of the American College of Allergy and Immunology, Nov. 12–16, 1988. Published in *Annals of Allergy*.

This double-blind American study was designed to determine the reliability of ALCAT Test results. Double-blind studies mean that neither researchers nor participants know who is receiving treatment and who is not. This method assures an impartial assessment of the participants.

This study was designed to test the accuracy of the ALCAT Test versus a traditional double-blind challenge with the same foods. (For the 58 ALCAT positive foods selected from the 19 subjects, 46 were positive on double-blind challenge [79.3%] and 12 were negative. Of the 56 ALCAT negative foods, 49 were also negative by double blind challenge [87.5%] and 7 were positive.) Overall correlation between the ALCAT Test and the double-blind challenge was 83.4%, suggesting the ALCAT Test was quite reliable in identifying unsafe foods in these sensitive subjects.

Høj, L. "Diagnostic Value of the ALCAT Test in Intolerance to Food Additives Compared with Double-Blind Placebo-Controlled Oral Challenges." Paper presented at the 52nd annual meeting of the American Academy of Allergy, Asthma, and Immunology, March 15–20, 1996. Published in *Journal of Allergy and Clinical Immunology*, Vol. 97, no.1, part 3, Jan. 1996.

This Danish study was designed to determine whether the ALCAT Test could consistently detect intolerance to food additives. Using 26 randomly chosen patients with known food additive intolerances, 76 food addictive challenges were done using the double-blind technique. The ALCAT Test predicted negative and positive reactions with 95% accuracy.

————. "Food Intolerance in Patients with Angioedema and Chronic Urticaria: An Investigation by Rast and ALCAT Test." Paper presented at the XVI European Congress of Allergology and Clinical Immunology, Madrid, Spain, June 25–30, 1995. Published in *European Journal of Allergy and Clinical Immunology,* Supplement No. 26, Vol. 50, 1995.

This test confirmed the effectiveness of ALCAT testing over Rast testing in determining the cause of angioedema (swelling) and urticaria (hives). This study also confirmed the importance of food sensitivities as a cause of allergic reactions and hives.

This Danish study used 52 patients to test the hypothesis of food intolerance being associated with chronic urticaria (itching) and angioedema (whelps). When patients' individual diets consisted of foods to which (according to the ALCAT Test) they showed no sensitivity, there was complete remission of both angioedema and urticaria in 45 patients, remission of angioedema but not urticaria in 5, and failure in 1.

Kaats, G., D. Pullen, and L. Parker. "The Short-Term Efficacy of the ALCAT Test to Facilitate Changes in Body Composition and Self-Reported Disease Symptoms: A Randomized Study." *The Bariatrician,* Spring 1996.

This Texas study evaluated the benefits of supplying dieters with information about their food sensitivities.

Subjects had body composition measurements taken and were given a disease symptom questionnaire. They were then separated into two groups, with one group being given a diet plan based on their ALCAT results. The other group (the control group) was asked to pursue a weight-loss plan of their own choosing.

Results showed the ALCAT group lost significantly more pounds, body fat percentage, and body fat weight than the control group. The ALCAT group also reported improvements in all 20 symptoms listed in the disease symptom questionnaire.

Pasula, M., and S. Puccio. "Multiple Pathogenic Mechanisms in Food Sensitivity Reactions In-Vitro." Presented at the 4th International Symposium on Immunological and Clinical Problems of Food Allergy, Milan, Italy. Nov 5–9, 1989. Published in the proceedings.

This study evaluated the multiple pathogenic pathways involved in food allergy reactions. Whole blood from nine food-sensitive asthmatic patients was incubated with each extract, and immunoglobulin levels were measured. Significant changes in one or more immunoglobulin and complement component occurred in every patient to one or more foods. The ALCAT Test was shown to be effective in identifying these food sensitivities.

Sandberg, D., and M. Pasula. "A Comparison of the ALCAT Test for Food Reactions Amongst Two Population Subgroups." Presented at the 45th Annual Congress of the American College of Allergy and Immunology, Los Angeles, Calif. Nov. 12–16, 1988. Published in *Annals of Allergy.*

This study was designed to test whether the ALCAT Test can discriminate between a healthy group and a group with food allergies. The study used a control group of 25 healthy young athletes with no history of food sensitivities and an age-matched group of 25 young people with suspected food sensitivities. Of the 225 reactions observed for each group, the healthy group had a total of 5 positive reactions compared to 45 reactions for the patient group.

Solomon, B. "The ALCAT Test: A Guide and Barometer in the Therapy of Environmental and Food Sensitivities." *Environmental Medicine,* Vol. 9, No. 2, 1992.

This study reviewed 172 individuals one to two years after they began diets based on the results of their ALCAT Tests. An independent reviewer asked patients to evaluate the effect of food elimination and/or allergy shots on their symptoms on a scale of 1 to 10.

Results confirmed the value of the ALCAT Test results and elimination diet in alleviating symptoms such as migraine, sinus congestion, irritable bowel, gastrointestinal reflux, arthritis, asthma, fatigue, obesity, and eczema.

Steinman, H., M.D., Department of Clinical Science and Immunology, Medical School, University of Cape Town, South Africa. Unpublished study, 1997.

In this South African study, 12 patients were tested using the ALCAT Test for each of 50 foods. Each test was done in duplicate or triplicate samples, resulting in 94.4% reproducibility of the data. In addition to the high reproducibility of the scores, two patients suffering from gastrointestinal symptoms had dramatic improvement of their symptoms following an elimination diet constructed with the aid of the ALCAT Test.

ABOUT THE AUTHORS

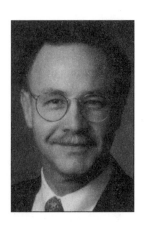

Rudy Rivera, M.D., has practiced medicine for 22 years in the fields of emergency medicine, anesthesiology, and bariatric (management of overweight) medicine. His interest in management of overweight and nutritional therapy stems from his own personal battle with overweight. Board certified in bariatric medicine, he currently is in private practice in Plano, Texas.

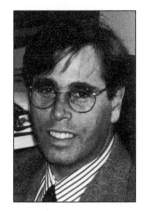

Roger Deutsch has been an advocate of alternative health care for the past twenty-five years. In 1973, he studied acupuncture in the United Kingdom and developed a strong interest in dietary factors related to health, as well as stress management techniques. In 1979, he launched a successful business career, becoming the co-founder and chairman of the world's largest international oil brokerage company, Amerex Oil Associates, Inc. In 1986, he founded AMTL Corporation (America Medical Testing Laboratories), which developed the ALCAT Test®, and has continued to serve as its president and CEO. He lives in Austin, Texas, with his wife Jenifer and son Jason.

INDEX

Index

Index

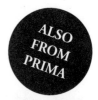
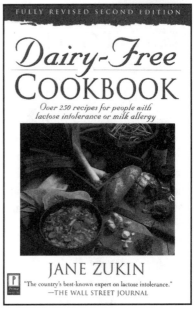

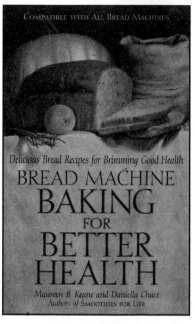

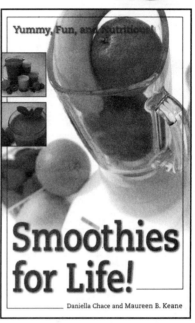

To Order Books

Please send me the following items:

Quantity	Title	Unit Price	Total
_____	**Dairy-Free Cookbook**	$ 15.95	$ _____
_____	**Bread Machine Baking**	_____	$ _____
_____	**for Better Health**	$ 14.95	$ _____
_____	**Smoothies for Life!**	$ 14.95	$ _____
_____	_____	$ _____	$ _____

<table>
<tr><td rowspan="10">

*Shipping and Handling depend on Subtotal.

Subtotal	Shipping/Handling
$0.00–$14.99	$3.00
$15.00–$29.99	$4.00
$30.00–$49.99	$6.00
$50.00–$99.99	$10.00
$100.00–$199.99	$13.50
$200.00+	Call for Quote

Foreign and all Priority Request orders:
Call Order Entry department
for price quote at 916-632-4400

This chart represents the total retail price of books only (before applicable discounts are taken).

</td></tr>
</table>

Subtotal $ _____

Deduct 10% when ordering 3–5 books $ _____

7.25% Sales Tax (CA only) $ _____

8.25% Sales Tax (TN only) $ _____

5% Sales Tax (MD and IN only) $ _____

7% G.S.T. Tax (Canada only) $ _____

Shipping and Handling* $ _____

Total Order $ _____

By Telephone: With American Express, MC or Visa,
call 800-632-8676 or 916-632-4400. Mon–Fri, 8:30–4:30.
WWW: http://www.primapublishing.com

By Internet E-mail: sales@primapub.com
By Mail: Just fill out the information below and send with your remittance to:

Prima Publishing
P.O. Box 1260BK
Rocklin, CA 95677

Name _____

Address_____

City _____ State _____ ZIP_____

American Express/MC/Visa# _____ Exp. _____

Check/money order enclosed for $ _____ Payable to Prima Publishing

Daytime telephone _____

Signature _____

$25 Discount for the ALCAT® Test

This coupon entitles you and any family members (same address and last name) to **save $25** on the price of an ALCAT Test.* Please enclose this coupon with the blood and requisition form.

Contact AMTL for details by phone:
(954) 923-2990 or (800) 881-2685
or fax: **(954) 923-2707.**

* Test must be for 100 or more determinations. Good only in the U.S. and Canada.